AF574158

GIVE IT TIME

To ANNE, my sister,
who encouraged me to write this book.

GIVE IT TIME

An Experience of Hospital 1928–32

BELLA ARONOVITCH

Preface by Professor Brian Abel-Smith

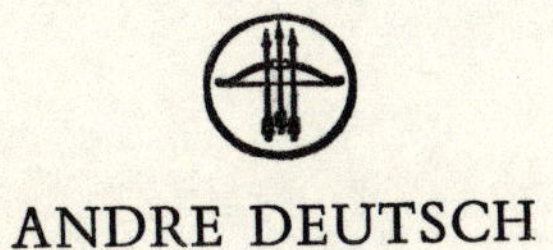

ANDRE DEUTSCH

First published 1974 by
André Deutsch Limited
105 Great Russell Sureet London WC1

Printed in Great Britain by
Ebenezer Baylis and Son Ltd
The Trinity Press, Worcester, and London

ISBN 0 233 96522 X

Preface

Much has been written about hospitals in the inter-war period by doctors, nurses, administrators and social reformers. But remarkably little has been written by patients. Bella Aronovitch's account of four years in five different hospitals is richly authentic and deeply moving.

Miss Aronovitch called in to see me about two years ago carrying a bulky and rather untidy manuscript. With an humility which I found embarrassing, she asked me whether I could possibly spare the time to read her book to see if anything could be made of it. I took it home and started to browse. I went on reading until late in the night. I was captivated. The only book I could compare with it was Thompson's *Larkrise to Candleford.* It had more in common with this than John Vaizey's *Scenes from Institutional Life*.

The period about which she writes (1928-1932) was a critical period of transition in hospital history. The London County Council took over responsibility for the workhouse infirmaries and started the process of upgrading. It was by no means uncommon for the patient who had failed to respond to treatment in the voluntary hospital to be dumped, like young Bella was, into the infirmary and even ultimately transferred to the House. Bella tells how she escaped ultimate rejection to the workhouse by a hair's breadth.

Bella suffered the slights of being an object of charity with remarkable tolerance. Her story is so much more powerful for the absence of self-pity and the placid acceptance of every slight she had to bear. But she observed everything and felt everything —the pain, the arrogance, the disregard by hospital architects, doctors and nurses for so many of the patient's real needs.

Not all that Miss Aronovitch describes has been swept away.

Many of the buildings are still there—if refurbished and refitted. Despite the National Health Service some of those who work in hospitals retain the attitudes and traditions of forty years earlier. How often are patients and relatives denied the knowledge to which they have a right? How often do doctors and nurses still carry on conversations across the patient—as if the latter were an inanimate object? How many sisters become autocrats in their own wards, distribute arbitrarily both punishments and rewards and expect patients to tolerate more pain than is necessary. Those who work in hospital have a special need to read this book, to listen to the patient's point of view and ask themselves whether they and their colleagues are really putting the patient first.

Younger people today take the National Health Service for granted—particularly the right to hospital care. This book explains part of the reason why a health service was needed. Hospitals could not be left in the hands of charitable donors and localised under-financed public authorities. A hospital system must be planned to ensure that the right care is made available for each patient. It should not have been left to Bella's mother to find the right surgeon and beg him to do his best to save her daughter from a life in a home for incurables. But the provision of the right facilities and a method of directing the right patients to them is not all that is required. The patient's voice must always be heard—loud and clear. Bella's message is as important today as it was forty years ago.

BRIAN ABEL-SMITH
December 1973

I

WHEN I first started work I was apprenticed to a furrier in that part of London known as 'The City', where I worked from 8.30 a.m. to 7 p.m. and until 1 p.m. on Saturdays. There was one hour's break for lunch between 1 and 2 p.m. and also a full half-hour tea break between 4.30 and 5 p.m. Although we had tea every morning there was no pause except on Saturday morning, when we stopped work for a few minutes. It was part of my duty to make all this tea which totalled more than seventy cups each day and for which each worker paid threepence a week. Many workers at this firm, as a form of banter, spent considerable time calculating the sum total for the tea, as against the outgoing expenses involved buying tea, milk and sugar. It was finally concluded I was making enormous profits and would most certainly retire on a large fortune, as a result of the huge sums of money which accrued to me.

I earned seven and sixpence when I first started and had graduated to one pound by means of half-crown increases given somewhat grudgingly at irregular intervals. From this one pound my mother allowed me five shillings each week for fares, two lunches out and sundry odd expenses – the rest of my wages went into the household money.

At the beginning I mentioned the word 'apprenticed' which, in this context, needs an explanation. Many young people were then apprenticed to a trade in this way, some with formal indentures drawn up, wherein most employers paid as little as possible, whilst giving an undertaking to teach the trade to the young person concerned. The length of the apprenticeship varied between different industries and was usually three years in some light industry and as many as seven years in printing and other trades. In my case there was a verbal agreement between the employer and my father which held good. Along with many other school-leavers in similar situations I spent many months running errands, was at the beck and call of everyone and spent a large part of my time at work making the everlasting tea and washing the cups. (There were no saucers, so that if it was not elegant, it was at least labour saving.)

There were no serious complaints during the next two years or so that I worked, except on my side, about the lack of specific timing for the increases. The employer paid me little but did not give anything to those who taught me, for most part highly experienced workers, who were expected to put on a plate a lifetime's experience for which they never received a penny extra, other than their basic rate of pay. I merely mention this in passing as one of the various forms of exploitation that were common practice.

It was at this time that I started to feel ill. I worried about what might happen in the event of a break in my earning capacity, since our home circumstances were nearly always precarious: more especially as my father, who was an asthmatic, had been particularly ill that winter and unable to get about very easily. I did not appear to have spectacular symptoms of acute illness or perhaps I chose to ignore what was happening. This seemed to be the pattern: during the morning I did not feel too bad, though by the afternoon I was in some difficulty and became progressively more ill during the night. Again, in the morning I seemed to improve. I did not want to have time out as no worker was paid for time lost through illness, so that I was just worried about the short-term aspect, since the idea of a long illness never crossed my mind. Ever since I can remember I have had a Micawber-like approach to life and believe the next day will be better. After more than two weeks of 'feeling under the weather' as the foreman described it, this philosophy asserted itself and I did nothing – believing the next day I would feel better, though by this time I found it hard to pretend, even to myself, that there was not something very wrong with me. I managed to go to work every day until a certain Monday in February 1928, when I finally had to give up. I had worked all the morning and did not leave the firm until the lunchbreak. My employer, who was a well-to-do man with an established business, not only never again sent me any money, but did not even pay me for the half day which I managed to work.

When I left work at lunchtime, I first decided to go home, then changed my mind and went instead to the outpatients' department of a hospital, in the hope that the doctor there might suggest something to make me feel better. I remember cutting through one of the various alleyways off Aldersgate Street which was my usual homeward route and walking slowly towards the bus stop. I had not gone very far when I stopped to rest. It was at this point I took the decision not to go home and turned off in an entirely different direction. This hospital was chosen at random. It was not easily accessible or near my home. Frankly, I do not know why I chose it, except that it was one of the smaller hospitals since I was always afraid of the very large ones, although I had never been in one.

Thus began an illness which started as acute appendicitis and continued for more than four years.

Although I felt very ill generally, I was not in severe pain when I arrived at the hospital. I did not consider myself ill enough to warrant asking the out-patients' sister if I might see the doctor without waiting. As I was the very last patient, I waited two hours.

This department was the Casualty, as distinct from the main out-patients. The doctor in charge was a young man who looked as though he had so many things on his mind at the same time, that he seemed slow and withdrawn. A large number of people were seated on wooden benches waiting to see him. He answered numerous questions from Sister and other members of the staff, and at intervals was called away. When the doctor returned he continued to see the people in rotation who were seated outside his surgery. It was all very slow – time did not seem to matter.

While waiting I watched the other people, particularly a man with his arm encased in heavy plaster. Having seen the doctor the man came out and sat in a small side room. Someone who looked like the hospital porter arrived carrying a medium-sized saw and as he entered the side room, the door of which was open, I watched with alarm as he proceeded to saw through the plaster on the man's arm. I had great misgivings and fervently hoped that the man with the saw would know at which point to stop. When he finished sawing he cut through the padding under the plaster with a pair of shears, pulled the casing apart and lifted it from under the man's arm: he seemed very adept at this kind of work.

Eventually my turn came to go in and see the doctor, who by that time looked tired and irritable. He asked my name, age and address, which he entered on a sheet of headed paper and then said, 'What are you complaining of?' I replied, 'I haven't much pain but feel generally ill.' The doctor continued with some sarcasm, 'And where is this "not much pain" – I'll have a look at you.' In one corner of the Casualty room was a high, leather couch with an adjustable backrest, covered with a bright red blanket and almost hidden by a screen. The nurse whispered to me, 'Just pop round by the screen and slip your clothes down.' I was not quite sure how much clothing was supposed to come off or where the rest was to 'slip down'. However, I had plenty of time to work things out for the doctor had again been called away. I took off my coat and somehow wriggled out of my top clothing. I waited a while and put my coat round me as I started to feel cold. A few minutes later I heard the doctor return to the Casualty room and say, 'The girl, where is she?'

The doctor gave me a cursory examination and his attitude changed. He took my temperature and seemed a long time looking at the thermometer – then he took it a second time. He asked me how long I had been ill. I thought about three weeks. He said, 'Why didn't you come before?' I did not know exactly why; I thought I would get better. I then added gratuitously, 'I'm really very strong and athletic.' The doctor ignored that statement and sat down to write. He seemed to be writing a great deal – I presumed it to be about myself. I lay and waited, thinking he must say something sooner or later. Somebody else came over to see me (it was Sister) and speaking collectively said, 'We would like you to see another doctor – he's very nice and will be here soon.' Privately I thought one doctor sufficient.

By this time it had become dark. I felt restless and uneasy. No one at home knew where I was for I had decided to go to a hospital on the spur of the moment, having no real idea of what was wrong with me. My train of thought was interrupted by the arrival of the second doctor. He was a considerably older man, very tall and looked kindly. At first he asked the same questions as the other doctor and I gave the same answers. He then asked two additional questions. The first was 'Are you frightened?' I replied untruthfully, 'Oh no.' Actually I was terrified. The second question which I found even more surprising was, 'How did you get here – did you walk to the hospital?' 'Certainly I walked here.' I wondered whether the doctor realized I had been to work that same morning. Finally, he said, 'You will have to stay here for a few days, Girlie.' 'Impossible,' I replied. I would have to go home, explain what had happened to my mother and, if it was really necessary, I would return to the hospital later. The doctor answered very soothingly as though humouring a young child, 'Your mother will be told where you are, everything will be explained to her and there is nothing at all for you to worry about.'

Inwardly I started to panic. I thought of grabbing my clothes, dressing quickly and running out of the hospital. After all, I had managed to walk here and they could not keep me against my will. The truth was, with a flaming temperature and seriously ill, having once got off my feet I could hardly move.

I felt hemmed in by people. There were the two doctors whispering to each other, the outpatients' sister, a nurse and a porter with a trolley. The nurse and the porter lifted me off the couch between them and I felt myself being wheeled away into the unknown. I asked the nurse about my clothes. She answered, 'You won't be needing clothes for a while – your mother will be able to take them home when she comes to see you.' I had never been in hospital before. Angry, frightened, outraged at my clothes being seized, I felt myself a prisoner.

I seemed to be travelling miles on the trolley; actually I went to a lift at the far end of the hospital and into a second floor ward. It was a relatively small ward with twelve beds and looked brighter than I had anticipated. Here I was handed over to the staff-nurse, who helped lift me off the trolley on to a bed near Sister's table. I learned afterwards that emergencies were always placed in beds near Sister's table, so that the night-nurse might more easily see what was happening. The table was quite small and stood halfway down the ward. On top stood a large lamp, the light of which was muted by a dark green cover over the shade. At night, it gave the surrounding area a weird, ghostlike effect. I then watched with smouldering indignation as the staff-nurse unceremoniously tied my clothes into a bundle and handed the bundle to the junior nurse, with instructions to give it to my visitors to take home. Separated from my clothes I felt, so to speak, a captive, resigned to an unknown fate.

The only thing that could divide one patient from another in the ward was a set of three screens, which the nurses were perpetually carrying up, down or across the ward. These screens had to be lifted as they did not have wheels. They served as the only privacy for patients and, in cases of death, were the only dividing line. The simple idea of curtains round each bed did not reach some hospitals until years later. When my mother came to see me I was screened off from the rest of the ward.

Mother looked worried and told me I would have to have an operation. This was the first time the word had been mentioned to me. All the previous feeling of fear and panic returned more acutely than before. However, I tried to appear unconcerned and urged my mother to speak to someone to see if anything was possible without an operation, since I was certain I was not as ill as all that. Mother told me she had already suggested this and nothing else could be tried.

Suddenly I changed the subject and said to Mother, 'How did you get to know I was here?' Mother then described to me how a young policeman had called at our house and told her he was attached to the local Station. 'A very nice young man,' Mother continued, although she wondered where the conversation was leading and what was the real purpose of his visit. The policeman continued by asking Mother whether she had a daughter – here he mentioned my full name – that I was in hospital and would she go to see me. 'I left everything and here I am,' were the final words of this report. The nurse then appeared from behind the screen and suggested Mother should go; as she said goodbye I felt my last bastion had fallen and that I was completely and utterly alone.

2

THAT was how it all began. The story of nearly five years of illness and its aftermath, which lasted much longer. On that first night in hospital when my mother came to see me and I felt 'utterly and completely alone', it was not merely because I was in the hands of strangers when she left, but that I was severed from my family, friends and work, to which my chances of returning were, had I known, almost nil. Although it happened to me the writer, many others were involved, not least my parents, my sister and brother. If I am asked who was the central figure? Whose role was the more important? I do not think I can readily answer 'mine', for the role my mother played seemed no less vital. In circumstances not of her making, in a chain of events no one could have foreshadowed, the part she played in changing a hopeless situation into its opposite deserves a rightful place in this story.

In recording the events which happened to me during this illness, other aspects seemed pushed into the background. For example, my father seems a shadowy figure. Actually this was not so. It appeared this way because he was already a dying man when I became ill, so that my contact with him became progressively less over the years, since the journey to come and visit me in hospital was too much for him. I always had news of him and wrote regularly until the final year, when I got better and he died. Recollections of my father have always been vivid.

In trying to present a more detailed account of my father and mother I cannot isolate them from their respective families and friends who, each in their own way, played a part in shaping all our lives. A considerable amount of what I am about to relate happened before I was born, for my parents were glad not to have started a family quickly because they could not afford one.

I know many of the details as my parents used to tell my sister and myself a great deal about their early life. They would talk about themselves spontaneously and naturally – we children loved listening.

My parents emigrated to this country from Minsk in Russia about 1903. They had recently married and were both very young.

My father, who was a radical and progressive, came from a poor family. He was a man of many talents with an extensive knowledge of Hebrew, which he was able to translate rapidly verbatim. He read voraciously in Hebrew, Yiddish and later in English. Ostensibly Russian was his native language. Both my parents had a working knowledge of Russian, for it was in that language they would converse in order to maintain a really private conversation. Although there is an extensive Russian literature, few of the poorer classes had a really sound knowledge of that language due to widespread illiteracy and lack of schooling. What applied to the people as a whole applied even more to the Russian-Jewish community who were obliged to live in set areas and for most part cut off from cultural contact with the rest of the community. I do not know a great deal about my father's family, other than he was a son by a previous marriage and that he had two half-sisters. I possess a most charming photograph of his mother, with whom my parents lived for a short time after their marriage. My mother always recalled her mother-in-law in terms of great affection. However, my father possessed a basic inadequacy which, to the present day, I am unable to understand. He seemed quite unable to cope with the day-to-day struggle of making a living and, apart from one or two brief periods, could neither provide for himself nor for his family. Had he been a less intelligent and talented man, it might have been easier to comprehend why he was unable to make the grade on the most modest level. It used to be my mother's great ambition to have a small, regular sum of money each week so that she could rely on being able to pay the rent and have enough for food.

Mother was the second eldest of four – she had one sister and two brothers. Her father was a strictly religious man with a rigid outlook. He owned a fur and leather tannery which was quite a good business. Mother had a happy and protected life with her parents until the age of fifteen though, within the next eighteen months, they both died. That was the only period of security she was ever to know.

My mother had an unusual name – Zelda. I rarely came across the name so that I was intrigued that the wife of the writer Scott Fitzgerald, who was a South American belle, should have been named Zelda. My mother was attractive. Of medium height, she had very long, dark straight hair with an unusual creamy skin without a trace of colour; she retained this rare skin beauty until her death in 1959. She did not have a particularly good figure, yet could wear the most ordinary clothes with an air of distinction. Mother was quick tempered and easily became excited and irritable, though she was able to laugh just as quickly. With her strong sense of the ridiculous and the bizarre, she was always ready for a laugh – very often at herself. By the time she was seventeen both her parents were dead, the family had split up and she was very much alone. It was at this time she met my father who never left her and they were married soon afterwards. I would like to be able to say they lived happily, but this I cannot do.

When my parents arrived in this country Father was unable to find work. My parents had really decided to settle in America and their stay in England was supposed to have been temporary, but they both made friends here and Mother had relatives, so they decided to remain in this country. Mother had quite a well-off family who had been established here for many years, and one of Mother's aunts offered my father a job. (I can just remember another of my mother's relations, an uncle, who was a sharp, peppery old man, with a large family. He heartily disliked all his four sons-in-law and claimed that he was much more attached to his five pomeranian dogs, one of whom was named Rosie, and who was able to walk a considerable distance standing on her two hind legs.) The offer of a job was really a gesture to help Mother, for the truth was, her relations did not like my father and considered Mother had made a hopeless marriage. My father started work, though he was well aware of the patronage behind the offer. He was a very quiet man and it took a lot to rouse him to anger; with a powerful inner life, he lived on two levels. Having earned his first week's money, which was a gold sovereign, he spent half of it on getting himself a good tutor in order to master the English language. He was extremely pleased with himself and urged Mother to take lessons with him, since the tutor said he would not charge much more for teaching two.

Mother was speechless when she heard this proposition. Having recovered herself, she pointed out one or two details about being behind with the rent and having to buy food. When my father replied that it was much more important to master the language, Mother was convinced she had married a madman. Her relatives were furious about the way my father was using what they stressed was their payment of a sovereign each week and took him to task concerning his behaviour. Now it was difficult if not impossible to quarrel with my father so, after three weeks, he quietly left Mother's relations and was once more out of a job. Father gave up the job but not the tutor, with whom he made an arrangement to continue his lessons and the tutor agreed to wait for payment.

Years later Mother admitted she had not understood the importance of what my father was trying to do when during the very first weeks he was in this country, he quite rightly placed the mastery of the language first, for Mother never did properly grasp the grammar and structure of English.

When Mother was a girl at home with her parents they had a tutor to teach Russian, Hebrew, the Scriptures and arithmetic. The pace of tuition was leisurely and irregular with no sense of urgency and no pressure to reach minimum standards. As I have already said, the majority of Russian people were illiterate and it was even more difficult for the Jews to attend Russian schools because of the Numerous Clauses Act which limited the intake of Jews to a minute percentage. Mother told me about her aunt who lived in St Petersburg and had two daughters having higher education. This was a rare circumstance, since Jews had to have special permission to live in the capital and many other important cities. Permission might be granted for two reasons: either for those who had served for twenty-five years in the Tsar's army, or for those with very special skills who happened to be needed in the big cities. Mother also described a visit she made to this aunt as a child of twelve years old. She stayed in St Petersburg a month and in order to do this, special papers had to be obtained through the authorities which took weeks of negotiation. This system of making it difficult to move around obtained for everyone.

Mother had worked for a time. She had been apprenticed to a couture dressmaker since this was considered a genteel occupation for girls. Mother could sew beautifully and this was one of the things she missed doing most when her eyesight failed almost completely.

As my father was without a job he continued to study English. The situation with regard to food and rent must have been desperate. By temperament he was the exact opposite of Mother—although he was no less worried, he tended to keep things to himself. In spite of difficult circumstances my father always attracted people towards him and made lifelong friends. In fact, some might well be described as disciples since they came to the house for years on end merely to converse with my father. Among these was a man named Mr Rogat who knew me from the day I was born. He always seemed to me a very old man, which was merely due to the fact that he was prematurely grey. When my father first came to London he became acquainted with Mr Rogat and this was one of the many friendships which lasted until my father died. At every available opportunity he would sit with my father, even during the winter months, when he was often quite unable to carry on a sustained conversation because of his acute asthma. Mr Rogat continued to come and see us for years after Father died, though I always suspected he came more from habit for, so far as he was concerned, there was no substitute for the discussions he had with my father. Mother told me that Mr Rogat was as distressed as any of us in the family at the premature death of my father and did what he could to help her during this crisis period.

Another of my father's friends was a small, dapper man, who was a craftsman cabinet maker: he could make anything out of wood. My sister and myself used to be fascinated by a cane he carried which he fashioned himself. This cane, I remember, was made from a light-coloured wood and had an elaborate ivory handle which unscrewed to reveal a long, glass, inner tube, fitted into the outer wooden case of the cane. He only once removed the glass inner tube for us to see, for he was afraid it might break. Apart from being a very clever craftsman, he also had a bent for philosophy. His conversations with my father sounded like an unknown language to me and while this was going on his wife would be having separate talks with my mother about day-to-day problems. As a sign of the times, I clearly recall one thing he said. He was one of the fortunate people in a very good job with regular employment, though he had no illusions. Notwithstanding he had worked for the same firm for many years, I remember his telling my parents that he continued to remain a master craftsman only for so long as the firm existed and should anything happen to the firm, he would never again have similar status – such jobs were few and far between.

Mother decided to try and get some work on the strength of her previous short training as a dressmaker. Her first job was with a tailor who made suits for military bandsmen. The jackets of these suits were long, bright red, heavily embroidered with braid, and all the way down the fronts had about a score of hooks and eyes sewn together as closely as possible. It was Mother's job to sew the hooks and eyes in very securely because of the weight of the jackets. There was a piece-work system and Mother was paid a penny farthing for each jacket. (The year was about 1903–4. There is now no monetary denomination as small as a penny farthing. This was one example of the sweated labour conditions prevailing in many industries, which led to the formation of the first Wages Councils by the Government of 1909.) Not being used to such a heavy form of tailoring, Mother's hands became very swollen and she earned next to nothing. It was hopeless, as my father pointed out. She left that job and found another making blouses.

As labour conditions change, so does fashion. Since labour was very cheap and plentiful at that time, the style of blouses was very elaborate. These were, of course, blouses for high fashion. Made out of expensive silks, the patterns were most complicated. Mother said that although each blouse was different, for most part they contained a yoke, frills and scores of tucks, with the most elaborate sleeves. A considerable amount of work on them was done by hand. The first day Mother went to this new job she did not return home until 10 o'clock at night. My father became really worried. Mother eventually arrived and explained the normal working day was from eight in the morning and there was no fixed time for leaving off work, as that depended on how much there was to do.

The next night Mother did not return until 11 p.m.! This was more than my father could stand. Outwardly calm, though really in a raging fury, he went round to this firm on the third night and demanded to see the employer. In fact, he burst into the workroom, told Mother to get her hat and coat and took her home. It seemed the employer took fright at this scene and he told the other girls to go home as well. Mother never returned to the job. A short time after this my father managed to find a job in the fur industry which was seasonable, unreliable, with long hours and bad pay. As a child, I well remember seeing my father at weekends only when he was working, for he went to work before I was up and returned home when I was in bed.

Although my parents were without children for several years after their marriage eventually my sister was born, next myself and lastly our brother, who was the most wanted and loved of all babies, since he was the only male. We were now a family of five though the early pattern continued – my father was unable to make a living. He tried business and was not so much no good at it, as he was fundamentally uninterested in making money. Unlike Mother, he was a poor judge of people and believed only good of everybody. Neither could he bear to be shut away in a factory. How deeply I came to sympathize with him over the years and to understand this desire to be free from the monotony and the perpetual surveillance. In all fairness to my father there were one or two periods when he did make some money, though this was never enough to tide over the lean times. He was asthmatic, and this condition became progressively worse each year. He was in the army during the first world war and served for some time in the Labour Corps. Having contracted pneumonia badly this, coupled with asthma, made him very ill and he was discharged just before the 1918 armistice. My father lived for some years after the war though how he managed to survive the winters was a miracle. The doctor once told him that if he went to live in South

Africa and did only very light work, he would live a lot longer, to which my father made no comment – there was nothing to say.

One morning he died quietly without giving anyone much trouble so far as illness was concerned for Mother was in the same room with him and had no idea he was dying. He died whilst I was in hospital, leaving the rest of the family virtually destitute. I will return to this episode towards the end, as the death of my father coincided almost exactly with my coming home from hospital for good – in this forlorn way his life ended when mine had begun anew.

Yet from early childhood, my father left a deep and lasting impact. How was it he was able to exert such an influence on our lives? The reason was this. He was a true intellectual and in other circumstances might have gone far. Always well informed he knew a great deal about literature since there was hardly a classic he had not read and was able to discuss in detail, moreover he was highly articulate. As I have said, when I was young my parents and more especially my father had many friends who came to see us at week-ends. They would not drink a cup of tea to which they had not contributed. And what did everyone do for hours on end? They discussed and debated literature, poetry, politics, the trade union movement, social conditions and current affairs.

My sister and I used to sit on the floor and just listen. We regularly heard the cut and thrust of debate – the different angles on the same subject sometimes reduced to hair-splitting arguments. Much of this was right over our heads for we were far too young, yet much was retained even if we did not understand, for after the discussions by the grown-ups, came the secret discussions between my sister and myself. Sometimes odd confusions would arise as, for instance, I remember one day hearing the name 'King Lear', and was puzzled for a long time as to how a feminine Bible name such as 'Leah' could be equated with a king. My sister, who usually provided satisfactory answers to the most knotty problems, seemed unable to explain that one. The fact remains, however, that very early in life we heard the names Shakespeare, Dickens, Ibsen, Emile Zola, Tolstoy, Sholem Asch, Sholom

Aleicham and a host of others. Mother also listened and joined in the discussion often to disagree.

We did not go out very much and when we did it was not very far afield. There was one exception. My parents had two sets of friends both living at Barking, which was then very open and more like the country. Very occasionally we made a whole day's outing there, where we would divide the time first at one friend's house and then the other. Two things stand out very clearly in my memory about those friends. The first were a childless couple and I remember the woman for her most beautiful speaking voice and the other family because an aged grandmother lived with them, a circumstance to which I gave a great deal of thought as there were no grand-parents in our family. Another reason we did not travel very far, might have been due to the fact that I was a great nuisance to take out because I suffered badly from travel sickness. I was all right for short distances after which I turned a delicate hue of green and started to vomit. This would usually be followed by an assortment of advice to my parents from the other passengers, ranging from the most advantageous part of the tram for me to stand and get the air, to what not to eat or drink before starting on a journey. We had no holidays, annual or otherwise. I never saw the sea until I became ill and was sent to a convalescent home when I was about twenty. My father had no relatives here at all, though we always kept on terms of great friendship with my mother's younger sister and eldest brother and his family. As I said earlier, Mother was one of a family of four of whom the youngest brother died first at the age of twenty-three and the eldest brother lived to a great age.

By way of entertainment we made regular visits to the Bishopsgate Institute to hear the then famous organist named Goss Custard. Here my father insisted on sitting in the front row and my mother complained bitterly that she could not enjoy the music because the vibrations of the organ made her feel ill. Both my parents were fond of music. Mother had quite a pleasing voice and would often sing. She was passionately fond of tenors to whom she would listen with wrapt attention when the opportunity arose. One day, in a rare confidential talk I had with Mother by the kitchen sink helping to dry dishes, she revealed to me that she would have loved to be married to an opera singer. I saw nothing amiss with such a proposal and thought it a pity that Father was unable to aspire to such a calling. Father appeared to have a preference for brass bands and organ music, for I think it was the only type of music that came his way. I was under five and had not yet started school when I first remember going to the Bishopsgate Institute to listen to those recitals which, by the way, were free. It was my first introduction to hearing professional musicians – I enjoyed it then and my enthusiasm has never waned.

We were great question-askers, especially my sister, and Father was wonderful at explaining things, and talked to us as though we were grown up. He never regarded questions as silly and had a knack of reducing apparently naïve questions to a proper perspective. My sister has always maintained that Father's explanations, together with the fact that we learned to read very early at school, formed the basis of an education which a lot of well-off children might have envied.

In the face of all this poverty one might have thought we children were unhappy. We were not. Although we possessed very few toys since there was no money to buy them, we played diabolo, marbles and gobs, all the hopscotch games and we had a wooden hoop. Our most prized possession was one pair of ball-bearing skates which Father bought us when he had a few spare shillings: these we shared and learned to use one skate each. All these games were not played at any time, but at definite seasons during the year. On wet days Mother used to put two chairs together for us to play 'shops'. She would give us scraps of food she happened to have in the house and take her turn as one of the 'customers'. Mother also had a deft way of folding towels and making them into dolls; she used to prop them up on chairs and we always resisted when the dolls had to be transformed back into towels. We were resourceful. My sister used to write plays and as she was always good at drawing, would cut out paper scenery and chalk the required scenes on it. All these plays were enacted with the help of our numerous young friends of whom there were droves. I had the unfortunate habit of forgetting either the words or the cue which made everyone very cross, though I was quick to point out the lapses were due to the fact that I was rather younger than the others, which usually restored the *status quo*.

The food situation was difficult. At a time when food was very cheap, we had many days on bread and cocoa. Mother used to inform us of this menu beforehand. As this went on intermittently for years we were used to it and never made a fuss. We children always came first so that if there was little for us to eat, goodness knows what my parents ate – if anything. The truth was our family was underfed.

Strangely enough we were quite well dressed, since my mother and her sister were both dressmakers. Remnant pieces of material were very cheap and they would think nothing of sitting up half the night and between them making my sister and myself a dress each. The suits for our brother and top coats for my sister and I were often made out of the grown-ups' cast-offs which Mother would unpick, wash and iron wet, which entailed such a lot of work that once this part was done, Mother regarded the rest as mere detail.

Looking back it was amazing how clever some of the emigrant women were with their hands. There were several living nearby and I especially recall two: a lady from Rumania (who made the most gorgeous toffee apples) and the other from Hungary. They both had large families and used to make the children's clothes in the same way as my mother and my aunt, though they had never worked as dressmakers. In those days there were no ready-made patterns available and everything was done by trial and error, with results that were most professional. My aunt and Mother were often consulted in an advisory capacity.

I cannot leave the neighbour who made the toffee apples without reference to her husband. She was a tiny slip of a woman and her husband a very tall man, well over six feet, with a shock of unruly red hair. They had a family of six children including a set of twins, with not more than nine years difference between the eldest and youngest child and lived in miserable, overcrowded conditions. This man could not stay long in one place – he had wanderlust. When we got to know them they had been to America, back to Rumania, lived all over Europe including a rather longer period in Paris and had also been to Ireland. As a child I can remember him suddenly taking a job in Scotland, whilst his wife and children remained living next door to our family. The man fancied himself as an organizer and was fond of telling his wife that the real reason she could never stop work, was because she never planned properly. Had she just planned the housework more efficiently, she would have plenty of free time. For long periods his wife took no notice at all of his gratuitous advice, though at intervals she turned on him with real venom and suggested he did the planning of the housework, laundry, shopping, cooking for eight people and he could then have all the free time. Oddly enough this husband and wife were fond of each other and rumour had it that he persuaded her to marry him in the face of the greatest opposition from his wife's family. It was simply that he had delusions about large-scale organization and, in a limited fashion, used to apply his theories to his wife's housekeeping: the situation lent itself to this kind of thing, since she always had more work than one person could possible manage. My mother listened carefully to the complaints the lady made about her husband's attitude to housework, which nearly always took place when she brought in some extra toffee apples she had made for my sister and myself. I recall Mother reporting some of these facts to my aunt and adding darkly, 'If I were married to a man like that – anything might happen!'

We children loved listening to Mother's stories about her childhood in Russia, which was a happy one. Time and again she told us about the nearby orchard full of cherry trees, where Mother and her friends could spend all day, pick as many cherries as they wished, for one kopec a day. Then there was the story of the near neighbour who had an only child, a little boy of four, who at that tender age developed a rooted dislike of his father and would never approach him. Mother said most evenings at bedtime the following scene was enacted: the child would kiss his mother good-night, take fond leave of their dog whose name was Merschik and flatly refuse to say good-night to his father. It seemed all the grown-ups shook their heads sadly not knowing where this unequal contest might lead. There was also the description of the little horse and trap which served for outings in the summer, and in winter was fitted with sleighs and decorated with bells. The horse always looked immaculate. His mane was carefully plaited with red tape, a task performed by a woman who helped in the house and lived with the family for years. Being a country woman she was considered an authority on animals. (My own recollections of this horse were so vivid that one day when we had a free drawing period at school, I managed to draw a recognizable sketch of this animal. When the teacher asked, 'Is this a horse you know?', I very proudly replied, 'Yes, teacher, I have known him a long time although I have never seen him.' The teacher, somewhat mystified by this reply, did not pursue the subject.)

To my young mind the most exciting story was the following one.

I have already mentioned the family business which was a fur and leather dressing factory, situated within walking distance of where Mother lived. Her father strictly forbade Mother to go near or inside the tannery. Having received this instruction many times, Mother's curiosity was aroused and she set about thinking out ways and means by which she might peep inside without her father's knowledge. She watched and waited quite a long time for the necessary opportunity to present itself, until one day she was able to do this. Mother said she was nine years old at the time and never forgot the shock she received when she entered the tannery. Once inside she was amazed and not a little frightened to see a group of men stripped to the waist, a pile of skins on the floor and the men jumping up and down on top of the skins. The men stood still when they noticed her, surprised to see a child watching them. Mother was rooted to the spot with astonishment then, giving a last quick look round, ran out of the tannery. (The dressing of fur and leather skins is an old craft. When my mother watched those half-naked men, they were softening the pelts and working in the natural oil by jumping on them, for mechanization of this process was introduced much later. This job has still to be done. A wooden contraption is used for the purpose which in fur dressing is called a 'Kicker'.)

Sometimes an event from Mother's early life would come to light by accident. When I was very young, we lived for many years in an old, dilapidated house with an underground kitchen, adjoining a scullery with a huge boiler, and a rambling garden with a large vine tree. Our garden backed on to the house of a family who were all deaf and dumb, with the exception of one member – a woman. There were two sisters and a brother all married to partners likewise deaf and dumb. All the deaf and dumb parents had children who were perfectly normal. It was a fascinating sight to watch the children chattering away among themselves but, when they wished to converse with their parents, their talking technique changed completely. They would first give their parents' clothes a sharp tug to attract attention and then, by a series of signs and word mouthing, make themselves clearly understood. I watched this method of communication for years and never had a clue as to how they made themselves understood. Now my mother succeeded in conversing with the deaf and dumb ladies for quite long periods. One day I asked her, 'How is it you are able to make yourself understood?' Mother explained, 'We had a deaf and dumb girl living with us at home for several years, so I learned to talk to her: we were both the same age – ten years old.' It appeared this deaf mute was a neighbour's child who had suddenly been orphaned. Without hesitation or further ado, my grandmother said she should stay with them until proper arrangements were made. She stayed five years, during which time Mother became adept at speaking and understanding sign language.

Many people, attracted by my father's original thinking and ideas, would comment on this to Mother who answered gloomily, 'It's all very well, but it does not provide meals or help pay the rent.' Mother, who was very down-to-earth, found it extremely irritating that my father was able to discourse on the most abstruse subjects, yet for the most part found it impossible to regularly provide the bare necessities for making a living. It was a question of priorities. Mother's life was one of perpetual uncertainty so she could hardly be blamed for feeling embittered. In so many ways my father was an unusual and highly original man, with his thinking far in advance of the times. He was also very considerate and would always get up extra early so as to help get my sister and me ready for school and do as many odd jobs as he was able. When Mother was thirty, she contracted tuberculosis very badly and had two long spells away from home as a result. She probably had this disease for a long time before it was eventually diagnosed and was the reason, among other things, why she always felt exhausted. When Mother became seriously ill and was taken into hospital my father arranged for our baby brother, then not two years old, to be looked after by a woman who also gave my sister and myself a meal after school. We went back home about 8.30 p.m. when my father returned from work and my aunt would also be there since she helped a great deal, notwithstanding that she too worked long hours at her job. We had two years of this kind of life.

My parents never lost their sense of humour, in spite of all the difficulties. Often a tense situation would start to build up and stop half way, because one or the other had seized on some humorous aspect and started to laugh. My father had a dry sense of humour. He would make some comment, which was followed by a second of silence, after which everyone laughed. Addressing my father, one day I heard my mother say, 'Shut the door, Morris, it's cold outside.' Father got up from his chair, closed the door, returned and said, 'There you are, now it's warm outside.'

Something which remained to the end with my mother was her literal interpretation of life – especially her attitude towards truth. It was childlike. Unfortunately, this approach deemed so quaint in children became an embarrassment later in life – not that Mother saw it that way. She sometimes made the most devastating remarks and I might say later, 'Did you have to say a thing like that?' Mother became quite pained and answered, 'Well, it was absolutely true.' Thus, through the truth and nothing but the truth, complicated situations arose and sometimes made Mother enemies. This attitude was also in many respects her strength, for it made her able to view a given situation as it really was and not as she might have wished it to be. Mother was nobody's fool. In her acute summing-up of people, her ability to concentrate on a difficult problem to the exclusion of everything else, until making a final decision as to what should be done she was rarely wrong.

To give a clearer picture of what my mother was like I will return once more to her early life.

The way in which the deaf and dumb orphan was received into the house, was an example of the free and easy atmosphere which prevailed in the house of Mother's childhood days in Russia. They kept open house for everyone. Mother told me they always had people in for meals. Every Sabbath there would be a minimum of three extra visitors; a stranger passing through the town and always some poor student from the Hebrew Seminar. This was probably the reason that Mother was always easy in her relationships with people and found no difficulty in breaking down barriers of shyness. Neither did different age groups bother her, for she just as easily entered into conversation with children as with adults. Contradictory as it sounds, Mother was not a very bold type, being very easily frightened and modest to a point of primness – it was simply that she had a natural approach to which most people responded.

Our landlord might have intimidated most people even if he had not uttered a word, although Mother conversed with him in her usual practical way and said afterwards, 'He's a very old-fashioned gentleman.' His very appearance was awe-inspiring and I used to gaze upon him spellbound, on the rare occasions that I saw him. The time would have been the early nineteen-twenties. The landlord was then well over eighty with a white beard and quite upright, though he moved slowly. He wore a brown Billycock hat, was enveloped in a large overcoat and since he refused to travel by car, travelled in a carriage drawn by two magnificent horses. Over his greatcoat he was always well wrapped up in rugs, accompanied by a manservant and the carriage driver. He owned a great deal of property some of which was very old and slummy, such as the house in which we lived. On rare occasions he arrived to take a look at some of his property, though there were clerks to whom the rent was paid and complaints written up in a huge ledger.

One of the landlord's clerks was quite a character in his own right. Aged about eighteen, tall, very earnest and always neatly dressed, he sat on a high stool with a leather-covered seat, in front of a large, open ledger in the cramped, dim, estate office, where the paint and woodwork was the colour of dark oak. I have seen more cheerful funeral parlours. The landlord's clerk took himself very seriously, though never more so than when he walked abroad to discharge certain other duties he performed outside the estate office. While on such excursions he always smoked a pipe and from time to time would stop opposite or outside the various properties belonging to his employers and gaze intently at the front walls of a house for quite long periods. It was difficult to divine his thoughts as he stood, pipe in mouth, staring at the fronts of houses. Although this action was quite passive, for he never spoke, it annoyed my mother intensely and one day after he had stood staring at our house for some minutes, Mother opened the door and asked him why he did this. It seemed at first the landlord's clerk did not intend to reply to Mother's question though, after hesitating, he took his pipe out of his mouth and said, 'I regard it as part of my duty to note, so far as possible, what is going on in any of the properties and, if necessary, to report back to the landlord.' Mother replied that she could tell him large numbers of things about the inside as well as the outside of the house which he could report back to the landlord, so that a few improvements might be made. To this he did not deign to reply: having replaced his pipe in his mouth, he moved on with dignity. In this curious way, the landlord's clerk lived in reflected glory of his employers.

The landlord's son treated his father with the utmost deference and would hasten to open the carriage door to help the aged man out, on the rare occasions when he came to look at the house in which we lived. The son might enter the house to check on the various faults for himself. Mother usually gave a long list of complaints about the state of the house, to which the old landlord and his son would gravely listen, say nothing and do only the barest minimum when a situation arose that constituted a danger. For example, one day the wall one side of the garden completely collapsed of its own accord. The landlord merely sent to collect the bricks and partly clear away the rubble, though the wall was never again rebuilt or a substitute provided. It was a wonder the roof of this house never caved in, for it was always leaking somewhere. I recall one severe leakage when the water almost poured down one side of the lavatory. Since negotiations with the landlord were always very protracted, Mother skilfully wedged an open umbrella under the lavatory cistern in the interim period.

To patch up the roof the landlord employed a man aged seventy-three, who told Mother he had worked for the old landlord since he was twelve years old. Mother thought it dangerous and inhuman that a man of his age should have to do outside roof work. One day she said to him, 'Can't the landlord find you an indoor job?' At this suggestion he chuckled and replied, 'No, I suppose I'll 'ave to go on doing this job until one day I falls orf the bloody roof.' Mother did not laugh at his reply. Her own life was beset with difficulties, yet she would pause to consider the plight of others. She always made him two lots of tea, one cup before he went up on the roof and another, with a slice of bread, when he came down. He told Mother that half a century earlier, the old landlord had bought up land for as cheap as half-a-crown an acre. I actually heard this conversation and, looking back, two things stand out: firstly, that it never crossed the mind of the old roof repairer he had any right to retire from work, and secondly, the nearest my mother could get to improve his conditions, was that he might be given an indoor job. Such was the thinking of those days.

I have one further recollection of the old landlord. We lived in the old dilapidated house belonging to him for many years. It was situated near a market to which Mother sent me one day to buy one or two items of shopping. Suddenly I espied the old landlord seated in his carriage, which had stopped by the side of this market. The landlord opened the carriage door, beckoned to one of the fruit stall owners, who responded at the double and was given an order. The stall owner returned carrying a considerable quantity of fruit which was stacked down beneath the driver's seat. During this fruit-buying transaction the driver did not get down from his seat. The stall owner shut the carriage door, respectfully touched his cap and the carriage moved on. Wild horses would not have dragged me from this scene. I stood and watched until the carriage was right out of sight and then bought the errands for Mother. All the way home I was greatly puzzled, for I visualized the old landlord living in a huge country mansion on a vast estate with orchards, flowers and vegetable gardens. The kind of thing I read about in story books. On my return home I told Mother what I had seen and we agreed that the old landlord must have bought fruit such as oranges and bananas which he could not grow himself.

How did our family manage to exist? Large numbers of working-class people lived a similar life to ours, so we were certainly not unique. We lived from day to day. There was no set pattern to our way of living, other than that of never having enough to manage on. Some weeks might be better than others. My father sometimes had a period when he earned regularly, though at the first signs of the work slowing down there was short time, or workers were laid off altogether. A favourite method used right up to the outbreak of the second world war, was to tell the worker to stay home for a time to see whether the work would increase, in which case the worker might get the job back. During this waiting period the worker was neither working nor officially unemployed. A few were fortunate and might be part of a skeleton staff retained, often at a lower rate of pay. Occasionally mother might do an odd job which came her way and thus earn a few extra shillings. Most of the time Mother was in a poorly rundown condition and often unable to get out of bed, though she hardly gave much attention to herself. Those employed on the buses or in the Post Office were much envied because they had regular jobs. We did well at school, yet our parents could not wait for the day when we were able to leave and start work, to contribute towards our keep. First my sister started work and then myself, though the amounts we earned were very small and irregular. For most school leavers there was little or no choice of work. Anything which was available was usually dead-end, soul-destroying work with little money and no prospects. As I have already described at the beginning, I started work for a furrier and was paid seven shillings and sixpence for a near fifty-hour week. From the very first week most of what I earned went towards the household expenses to help with rent, food and other bare necessities. There were times when Mother would wait for me to bring home my wages on Saturday and go straight out to do some shopping with the money. And when I say 'shopping', I mean basic food, which really went against the grain with Mother for religious reasons because it was the Sabbath.

In those circumstances, living as we did from hand to mouth, illness was a disaster which imposed a stranglehold on the family from which it was impossible to break loose. It was a vicious circle. Living under continual strain and uncertainty it was difficult to keep well. Not only parents suffered, but the perpetual agitation communicated itself to the children. For myself, right from the age of seven or eight I started to become aware of the difficulties which beset my parents. I was a very happy child for whatever else we went without, we had plenty of affection and were a stable, if not always united, family. From an early age, however, I started to think about the mysteries of 'making a living', which were discussed between my parents, sometimes none too amicably.

When I came out of hospital and having finally mastered the trade, I worked for many years for the same firm. Many of the people working there whom I had known for years, had a similar childhood to my own, a fact which was always an interesting topic for discussion. During one such discussion the foreman said, 'I was never a teenager – I went from childhood to manhood.' That was a very good description and applied to both sexes; it certainly applied to my sister, my brother and myself. There was somehow no time to indulge in being young.

My father was the kind of man he was because he could be no other. All else is wishful thinking. Mother spent most of her life trying to hold together a way of living that could not be anchored to anything reliable. No planning was possible. Yet, under those most difficult conditions, Mother succeeded in keeping the home together. With poor living accommodation this was no mean feat, for everything had to be done the hard way. However, it was the untimely death of our brother, an only son, which finally broke her spirit. Blind and very frail, she lived to be over seventy. In other circumstances I think she might have lived to be very old, for she had a tremendous zest for living.

Poverty is a relative term. I know people with property, covered by heavy insurance policies, living in conditions I would describe as very comfortable, refer to themselves as 'poor'. It is all a matter of comparison. Mother was a widow for many years and had to rely on me. When I came out of hospital I had all the difficulties of rehabilitating myself, which I will describe later in this story. However, for many years I did have a reliable job, where it is only fair to add, conditions of employment were higher than average. Mother was a wonderful manager in the home and we lived on the money I earned. To give an idea of monetary changes, my earnings rose from two pounds fifteen shillings a week when I first joined the firm, to twenty-two pounds plus, at the end of thirty-five years. (The 'plus' represents fluctuating bonuses.) The passing of the 1948 National Assistance Act improved conditions for Mother – a thing at which she never ceased to marvel. My mother was at the opposite end of the pole to some who believe everything is owing to them, for she believed that nothing was owing to her. As one of the meek she should have inherited the earth . . .

Mother came from a very religious background, something which remained an important part of her life. All the Holy Days were very dear to Mother – not that I did not enjoy them for they were something with which we had all grown up. She possessed some very rigid, departmentalized beliefs as, for instance, that Royalty were protected by special heavenly charter or, because the priesthood were endowed with much learning, it placed them on an elevated plane to ordinary people. And if some fell by the way, she maintained this did not invalidate the general principle. If it sounds inconsistent with my mother's other characteristics, such as her sense of reality and the fact that she was a good judge of people, I can only say she lived all her life with these apparently conflicting ideologies, which did not give her trouble or cause her to have any doubts. However, my father's rationalist and humanist approach to events gave me a kind of split personality with regard to religion. It became a circle which I tried to square. My sister and brother seemed less troubled by this for they took up a definite stand. I mention these facts because they cut across my relationship with Mother since what appeared plain and straightforward to her, was often anything but clear to me. Nevertheless, what disagreement there might be about the interpretation of ideas and events, there was one thing on which we were completely in accord – our dread of Institutions.

It was strange how Mother and I changed roles. All the years I was ill I relied on her implicitly, hoping she would find a way to get me out of hospital. Had Mother been a different kind of person this book could never have been written, since I am not the type to come to terms with being a perpetual invalid. Mother and myself were closely identified, for she intuitively understood what it meant to live for years in Institutions and often expressed her horror of such a life. Later, when she became blind and very dependent on me, there existed between us a complete bond on such matters. In spite of the difficulty of her being alone for long periods as my sister and brother were both married and away from home and I was at work all day – there was no question of Institutions.

A large number of people helped me get well; it would be insensitive and ungrateful of me to underestimate this factor. Yet, as this story will surely prove, no matter how obscure or grave the prognosis with regard to myself, no matter what host of domestic difficulties, behind all stood my mother, who was relentless and unceasing in her mission never to stop trying or think of giving up the fight to get me better. To this I have remained the living testimony and there can be no other evidence more telling or true. In order to trace how my mother accomplished this I return again to that first night in hospital when she left me in the ward after the first, brief visit.

3

After my mother had gone, the nurse came back and asked whether I wanted a cup of Bovril to drink. Having assured her that was the last thing I felt like drinking, she re-appeared with a large cupful of the stuff and urged me to drink it all, as it was very sustaining and good for me. I attempted a sip but had to leave it. By this time the night-nurse had come on duty. Like a ship in full sail, she was quite young but fat. With a pink-striped uniform, stiff collar and cuffs and a wide belt tight round her middle, she had a loud, fruity voice, red cheeks and looked the picture of health. She came through the screens and said very cheerfully, 'I will be giving you some castor oil presently. Don't worry, you won't taste it, because I am going to lace it with plenty of brandy.' By that time my resistance was completely worn down, so that when the night-nurse came back bringing the castor oil and brandy, I drank it as quickly as possible. Until then I had no symptoms of nausea or vomiting, which rather surprised the doctors: after struggling valiantly to keep down the castor oil and brandy, I vomited it up later. This, coupled with the after-effects of the anaesthetic, made me feel sick for the best part of a week. Hospitals had certain treatments for specific conditions which changed according to current discoveries, but were ritual and carried out regardless, until a new discovery was made.

Of all the advances in medicine, the improved methods of anaesthetizing must rank as amongst the most humane. To this day, over forty years later, I can clearly remember the devastating shock which the anaesthetic had on me at that first operation.

It is difficult to try and record what happened when I was actually taking the anaesthetic, because the feeling consisted of a series of physical reactions, visual sensations and sounds. Included also, though clearly separate, were the human voices. I was given the anaesthetic not in an ante-room but in the theatre proper. The place was so brilliantly lit, I found the light almost blinding. The anaesthetist came up behind me and said, 'Just keep this over your face and breathe normally.' I suppose he was referring to the mask, which I felt almost covered my face. The fumes of the anaesthetic came up in waves and seemed to be choking me. It was as though I were being forced to drink in much larger quantities than I could properly assimilate and I felt myself gulping. Again, the human voice said, 'Just take it easy and breathe away.' The night-sister who accompanied me to the theatre told me to hold her hands. I recall gripping her hands so tightly that I thought I must be hurting her – I relaxed my grip. She felt this immediately for she said, 'Don't let go of my hands,' so I increased my grip once more. The circular, coloured lights before me, in ever-increasing circumference, were very real. And then the sounds. These sounds were so clear that, years later, I was able to reproduce them on the piano. I do not know why these sounds came to me in the rhythm of music at first and then changed to the sound of rushing water. The pressure on my ears was unbearable. The human voice said, 'Do you think she's under?' I wanted to shout 'No' as I certainly heard what was said but the word was in my head and I was unable to speak it. Rapidly the sounds and sensations started to recede and become fainter – it was at this point that I lost consciousness. The time factor is quite fascinating – it seemed so long to me. Minutes or even seconds of misery or ecstasy can feel so entirely different as to make time seem an illusion.

Coming round after an anaesthetic, the feeling of time lost is impossible to estimate. I do not know whether other people did likewise but I invariably asked Nurse the time – usually the first words I was able to speak. Even when she told me I was never certain whether it was night or day and I used to check on this too. The climax of this maze of different feelings was the curious struggle to enter the conscious world. Once I had established the time, my thoughts always reverted to the last incident I could recall, though there was always this gap – this unaccountable nothingness. The time lost in being unconscious was like a kind of death.

After the first few days I became accustomed to hospital routine. It was the ward by night which seemed both eerie and fascinating. The shadows, the low voices, the dimmed lights, the sudden flash of a torch used by the night-nurse, all contributed to create this mystic atmosphere. Some nights the ward would be quieter than others, though there was always a restiveness. Several times I had seen people in evening dress, possibly friends of someone on the staff, standing and looking down the ward at night.

Many patients feel worse at night, and it was commonplace in all wards to hear the variety of sounds made by people talking in delirium, making the weird, frightening noises of people dying, or sounds by those who could no longer stand the pain.

Having mentioned pain, I also record with gratitude the changed attitude in all hospitals towards it. During all the years I was in hospital, the patients were expected to put up with pain as a matter of course. To illustrate this point I recall one occasion in particular. Along with everyone else in the ward, I was obliged to put up with a great deal of pain and one night it became so violent that sleep, or even keeping still, was impossible. The night-nurse knew of this and said that she would tell the night-sister when she came to do the round. Time seemed endless until, at long last, about one in the morning, the night-sister came to do the round. Her physical appearance was so unlike the usual nursing type, that I am able to recall in detail how she looked. With a petite figure, she had a pink and white skin and wore an elaborate goffered, lace cap, tied under her chin with a large, starched bow. Under the cap, her very fair hair was arranged in curls round her face with almost mathematical precision. No longer young, she was pretty in a doll-like kind of way and gave the impression of an early, middle-aged, Dresden china figure, that walked and talked. Sister stopped at my bed, asked me if the pain was *really* unbearable and said that if I found it impossible to sleep during the next few hours, she would ask the doctor to write something up for me. I neither saw the sister again that night, nor did I get anything to relieve the pain. Now this was not done in order to be unkind, it was simply the usual approach at that time; it was the way in which pain was regarded. There did not appear to be much available for the alleviation of pain. Everything had to be written up by the doctor so that even Mist. Aspirin was difficult to obtain. Things are very different now – the old attitude has changed. It is comforting to think that no one has to put up with pain as a matter of course.

A few days after this first operation I had a visit from the hospital almoner. She came into the ward carrying a huge sheaf of papers and looked terrifyingly efficient. Following a few minutes' talk with Sister she came over to me, made herself comfortable on a chair beside my bed and for the next quarter of an hour, her conversation consisted entirely of questions. She started with questions about my family. How many of us were there at home? Who went to work and who were still at school? How much did I earn when I went to work? How much rent did we pay? What was our total income from all sources? etc., etc. Now all the questions were the preliminary skirmishes leading to the final question, which was; could my family afford to pay towards my upkeep while I was in hospital and if so, how much? Having had a major operation I was stiff and sore with numerous stitches and draining tubes. Tied under my knees was a hard, uncomfortable pillow called a 'Donkey', and I was very tightly tied round the middle with an arrangement known as a 'many tailed bandage'. I found all those questions rather trying. However, I answered them truthfully and to the best of my ability. As the almoner left, she told me to be sure to tell my mother to call at her office next mid-week visiting day. She then double checked with Mother on the answers to all questions.

The almoner and her questions were part of a charity concept on which all hospitals were founded. At that time there were two main classes of hospitals: one, the Voluntary hospitals and the other, the Poor Law hospitals attached to the workhouse. There were also certain local government controlled hospitals for the treatment of fevers and tuberculosis. It was not until the following year 1929–30 that a very important law was passed and the Poor Law hospitals were taken over to be administered by the London County Council and County Borough Councils. Even after this law was passed, there was still an obligation on patients in all hospitals, for payment. The National Health Act of 1948 introduced a new concept for the first time, which removed the charity image from the health of the nation.

I recovered fairly well after the first operation. However, the incision did not close properly though I had been in hospital over two months. There were strange murmurings by the ward sister which I did not understand, about the wound being 'slow healing' and healing by 'second intention'. I was able to walk a little but the difficulty of the wound not healing persisted and it began to be evident that I could not get beyond this stage. The specialist then suggested I should have a second operation; as he cheerfully said, 'Just to clear things up.' I hardly received this news with wild enthusiasm, but philosophically decided that something else must be attempted, since I could hardly be very mobile with an open wound. Moreover, I faithfully believed in that mystique about the medical profession which is known as 'having faith in doctors'. Like numbers of working-class people I was overawed by the fact they wrote in Latin and carried on conversations among themselves which nobody else understood. They swept into the ward in a procession akin to Royalty. First came the specialist, flanked by his first-assistant on one side and the house-surgeon on the other side: some two paces behind were a varying number of students and this group were immediately joined by the ward sister. The rest of the nursing staff also became alerted. It seemed like a ceremony – a rite – I imagined I heard the sound of trumpets heralding the arrival of the sacred and the great, for they appeared to take on a God-like aura and be segregated from ordinary mortals.

It was about this time that my attitude towards the medical profession received a jolt.

Late one night a young girl was admitted into the ward as an emergency. Nothing happened until the morning when the specialist was due for his weekly visit. When he arrived he spent a while looking over her notes and making an examination and then said: 'You have an inflamed appendix and it will have to come out, Girlie.' The girl looked startled. He told her not to worry adding, 'It will not be a very serious operation.' The patient maintained it was impossible. The specialist gave her a bland, benevolent look and was about to move on, when she insisted it could not be true. He then paused and asked 'Why?' It seemed that the girl had already had an operation for the removal of her appendix some years previously. He went back and had another look at the girl, but did not say anything. Apparently it was such a good piece of surgery with the scar so faint, that the doctor had not noticed it. When the specialist had gone, the ward sister came up to the girl and said rather angrily, 'Why didn't you tell Doctor you had had an appendix operation?' The girl replied quite simply, 'He didn't ask me.'

After two weeks' grace and some ten weeks after the first operation, I had a second. It was much the same as the first, with my relief great at the knowledge that the anaesthetic was over. I was all set to become fit, well and back in circulation. In those days surgery was a much slower process and it was again six weeks before I was rid of the tubes and other paraphernalia. I sensed an air of concealment on the part of the doctor, though this was just a fleeting thought on my part and I did not worry.

When the specialist came to see me his face wore the usual sauve, calm expression which concealed the fact that anything was seriously amiss. Sister told him I was getting along fine. I regarded the fact that I was in hospital longer than anticipated as a mere nuisance. On the surface all seemed well. The specialist had a habit of coming into the ward at dinner time to do his round, whereon my half-eaten meal would be seized and taken back into the kitchen. When he and his entourage had gone and the dinner reappeared, I somehow never bothered about eating the rest of it. During one such dinner-time visit the specialist pointed out something on another patient's notes to the house-surgeon, who blushed to the roots of his hair. I was very curious as to why he was embarrassed and Nurse afterwards gleefully told me that he was weak on spelling and had written up ''flu' as 'flue'. This same specialist had other set habits. When he came into the ward he visited his own patients, of whom there were quite a number, and I noted that he shook hands very cordially with some of his patients. I wondered why this privilege was extended to some and not to others. Although his cases were all surgical, there was considerable variation as to the type of complaint, but I afterwards discovered that there was one thing which all the patients had in common with whom he shook hands – they had all paid him a private visit at his Harley Street surgery.

The result of the second operation was much the same as the first, that is, the incision did not heal beyond a certain stage. As part of the treatment it was decided to give me four-hourly fomentations, as this was much used before the discovery of antibiotics. The fomentation started off by feeling burning hot, after which it soon became lukewarm then, for most part of the four hours between one treatment and another, I had the feeling of being wrapped round with a cold, clammy blanket. This was continued for two weeks, day and night, making no difference whatsoever. Among other treatments, I remember being prescribed iodine – a few drops on a lump of sugar.

I did not mind this as I am fond of sweet things and the taste of iodine did not seem to trouble me. Nothing spectacular happened – the wound refused to heal. This situation continued for months, during which time the doctor was very fond of asking me whether I felt well in myself. I never quite knew how to answer that question. I felt I was being asked to subtract part of my body and give an account of what remained, for it seemed to me self-evident that I would have been much better without an open wound. This whole question of communicating with doctors has always appeared to me most difficult. As, for example, on another occasion the doctor said, 'Do you drink?' I replied by asking, 'Do you mean alcohol or just all fluids?' There was a pause – it appeared the doctor had not meant alcohol, though it certainly sounded as though he did.

A conspiracy of silence was being maintained by the doctor and the staff – if doubts existed, they were certainly not expressed either to myself or Mother. The sister on this ward rarely did any dressings though she occasionally looked on. During these viewing periods she was always sure so far as I was concerned, it was a question of time, a very short time and success was round the corner.

My mother became really worried. It seemed that she had spoken to the doctor several times and no more definite information emerged than, 'I will get better in time'. I believed the doctors knew exactly what was happening though, for their own reasons, decided not to tell.

I walked slowly and with difficulty. The deadly monotony of hospital routine made it hard to keep up morale and remain cheerful. There was nothing to look at. The walls of the ward were painted dead white and were completely bare. There was no decor, no pictures or ornaments of any kind. The only splash of colour during the day, were the flowers brought in by the patients' visitors.

In the evening, the bright red blankets showed when the white day quilts were taken off, folded, and slipped over the rail at the foot of the bed. Above all, there was nothing to do. In the days before radio was installed in all hospitals, the only communication with the outside world were newspapers, letters, books brought in by visitors and the official visiting days. There were no organized handicrafts, no library service, no mobile telephones; in short, there was nothing available to prevent people with long illnesses from sinking into depression. This, of course, did not affect short-term patients, as a short period of this kind of life often did people more good than harm. It was the long-term and chronic patients who felt all this so keenly.

The patients in the ward spoke to each other, usually the conversation consisting of a mutual exchange of symptoms. When the body breaks down this is quite naturally a cause of great concern to the person involved. It is surprising how the attitude of otherwise highly intelligent people is so absolutely concentrated on themselves, with the idea that what has happened to them is unique. I suppose every patient is unique in the same way that every person is, though many complaints fall into specific groupings with fluctuations that are not very marked. With the exception of two or three who had been there a long time, there was a complete changeover of ward patients about every three weeks. When new patients arrived, I could near enough guess the course of conversation with the different people. Some of the people in hospital were often very interesting, if they chose to talk about themselves other than their illnesses. Perhaps the example that follows is not very fair because of the extenuating circumstances, though it does demonstrate how difficult it is to gain any idea of what people are like when they are in hospital.

There was an attractive woman in the ward who had a leg

amputated and was in hospital three months. She gave me long and detailed accounts of how her illness started and how she arrived at a point where she had to agree to amputation. I understood and deeply sympathized, for the repercussions of this type of operation must be devastating. Just before she went home, having bravely fought to master the great difficulty of learning how to walk with an artificial limb, I asked whether her disability would greatly affect her work or hobbies. Unexpectedly she answered, 'Not in the least.' She then mentioned in passing, and for the first time, that she was a miniature artist and had many commissions awaiting her when she returned home.

There was no flexibility in the strict hospital rules laid down for visiting times. One and a half hours on Sunday afternoon and one hour on Wednesday afternoon were the official visiting times. Two and a half hours each week was considered quite sufficient, neither was there any allowance made for long-stay patients. Some of the ward sisters openly considered visiting times an unwarranted interference in the cycle of work and, as such, a nuisance. Sometimes the nurses were unable to get the ward work done in time, so that even these meagre periods were cut short by as much as twenty minutes and this time was always lost.

Officially the hospital allowed four visitors and not more than two at a time for each patient. As to how this rule was implemented depended on who was in charge. Sometimes the sister or nurse might spend the entire time policing the ward, to see that an extra visitor did not slip through the net. Other times a more tolerant nurse would be in charge and not bother to harry anybody. Both visiting periods were in the afternoon, so fewer people came on Wednesdays, since many who were working could not get away. There was not much time, so that occasionally visiting degenerated into a rapid question and answer session. When there was nothing to tell, visitors often expected startling revelations and waited on each word with bated breath.

The change in relationship with everybody in the outside world becomes strangely unreal. Many people have mentioned the fact that once in hospital even for a short period this change ensues, since a totally different code of behaviour is laid down and patients quickly become part of it. All the day-to-day stresses and strains of ordinary living are still there, though they take on a different dimension – they are somehow once removed. When patients enter hospital others take over and they make the decisions. The universe seems to shrink and in this curious metamorphosis the ward becomes the world. Those who brought news from the outside world were the most popular visitors, since ward patients live in a closed community and mostly feel very cut off. The most depressing time of all was after the visitors had gone – most especially on Wednesdays – as we did not see anybody until the following Sunday, which seemed an age away.

Very occasionally, visitors who had come a long journey, or could furnish an acceptable excuse, might be allowed into the ward to see someone, though this was at the discretion of the sister or charge nurse, and was not encouraged. Permission was usually grudgingly granted with the words, 'Well, you can go in for a few minutes this time.' The only exceptions to these rigid rules were for patients on the danger list, who were mostly dying and could have visitors at any time.

The economic situation in the early part of 1929 was bad. It was the beginning of the great slump which had already started in USA and swept across Britain, culminating in the disastrous unemployment of the early thirties. During my first year in hospital there was considerable unemployment, with devastating and demoralizing results. Sometimes a single incident will better demonstrate a situation than a great deal of explanation.

It was at this time that a young man came to the Casualty department of this hospital with his feet in a very bad state. He had walked from Liverpool to London and slept rough. Having worn out his shoes completely and thrown them away, he came out of the Casualty department with both feet heavily bandaged and wearing a pair of old slippers, which one of the nurses had found for him.

Now we in the ward came to know this story in the following way. There was a balcony running the entire length of the ward. In the early mornings, for want of something better to do, the patients who were up used to wander in and out of this balcony. We were all awake long before 6 a.m. Patients who were better, used to make an early morning cup of tea.

Breakfast was served by the day nurses at 7.45 a.m. It was the hours between six and eight that dragged, and it was then that the patients entered into conversation with the young man from Casualty. It was not easy to carry on a conversation as this ward was on the second floor, but they managed to get the story. The young man mentioned was one of a large family, none of whom was earning anything. The position in the provinces was worse than London with regard to unemployment. So it came about that the young man decided to try his luck in London, which he could reach in one way only – by walking. One of the patients was so moved by the appearance and the story of this young man that she asked him to wait. She stepped from the balcony into the ward, and suggested we might collect a few shillings for him. Everybody agreed to give something including the night nurses, though they asked us to do this quietly, as it might be misunderstood. One young woman, who was so ill she died a few days later, asked one of the patients to take sixpence out of her handbag and put it towards the collection. I remember the money collected came to nearly six shillings, which was wrapped in a piece of gauze and slipped through the iron railings of the balcony to the young man below.

Although I occasionally felt low, one thing was certain and that was I did not realize I had passed from the acute sick stage to the chronic sick. The realization of this fact did not come upon me until years later.

I had now been ill for almost a year and there was no sign of my getting better. The position seemed static. The way in which the hospital staff behaved made it impossible to obtain a perspective, since they said nothing: though these silences could be telling. Mother was often deep in thought when she came to visit me and I could tell she was mulling over the available facts, trying to think out what to do about me. One day she asked me whether the staff ever said anything amongst themselves about my illness that might give some clue as to why it seemed to go on and on. I told her the only thing I had heard was the specialist say to another doctor, with reference to myself, 'This girl has been here a long time – she was an emergency and I found she had the old-fashioned perityphlitis. I could not see much at the first operation because the organs were obliterated by pus.' Mother sighed and said she supposed things were not easy from the onset of this illness. There was obviously some discussion going on about me behind the scene because Sister tentatively suggested one visiting day, that there was a possibility of my going home for a while, 'To see how things worked out.' Mother agreed with this idea for her own reasons. The matter was not at all as simple as Sister's few, guarded, well-chosen words might have supposed. There was the problem of dressings, for the wound was by no means dry. The onus for solving this problem seemed to be left with Mother. It was vaguely suggested I should have a district nurse at home, and come up to see the specialist each week at the hospital Outpatients' department. I was unable to walk very much. This wound was curiously indrawn and contracted – I could stand up straight only by lifting my right leg well off the ground. The entire situation was far from satisfactory. However, Mother had other ideas, and in those circumstances no one could blame her for what she did next.

4

MOTHER decided to get another medical opinion about me and with this objective in view, she wanted me home. The alternative would have been to discharge myself from hospital though, on the face of it, there seemed little difference. However, it was by no means certain whether another surgeon would wish to do anything, or he might agree with just waiting. Mother discussed the matter with me at great length and we decided that I had gone as far as possible at this first hospital, where I had spent almost a year. All inquiries about myself met with one answer, namely, 'She will get better in time.' How long? Nobody would commit themselves. Once home, I never returned to that hospital. The attitude towards patients by the hospital authorities was then entirely different, for there were no further inquiries made about me. Under the present system the hospital Records Officer would have checked and helped to create a climate for more open discussion. Had I attended the Outpatients' department as was arranged, there would have been some form of follow-through. Sometimes it is best to do nothing. But when nothing was done and nothing was said, how was my mother to draw any kind of conclusion or reach any kind of decision – even if the decision meant it was better to just continue waiting? The difficulty of how much a doctor should tell, is as old as medicine itself and has always been a problem for the doctor's individual assessment. If the doctor did not regard me as mature enough to discuss matters, I did rely on Mother getting some explanation. She was very intelligent and even if there was little about which the doctor could be exact or reassuring – in short, if he did not know, some kind of explanation would have been preferable to the stereotyped reply, 'She will get better in time.'

Being home created many problems. I was only able to walk

with considerable difficulty. Out of sheer necessity I became proficient at doing my own dressings and making myself as comfortable as possible, though I was not without some theory, for I had watched the nurses do dressings since the second day I was in hospital. Nevertheless, it gave me a feeling of real joy to be home and once more part of the family, to be rid of the hospital discipline and be able to have visitors at any time. Deep down, however, there was a nagging feeling of apprehension not openly expressed, for Mother and myself both knew that my homecoming was a grave step – we had burned our boats; it was a point of no return.

Some of the things Mother was able to accomplish remain a wonder to the present day. She managed to get an appointment for me to see a consultant surgeon at another hospital. This surgeon was not just chosen out of the blue – he had a reputation for being very clever. Moreover, he had previously attended my young brother, so that he was not completely unknown to us when Mother went to the hospital where he was a consultant and asked his help. She faithfully told him all she knew about me. He agreed to see me at his own hospital first, obtain more information about me through my previous medical notes, and then decide what to do. It is only fair to add that he agreed to go into this without hesitating, for the entire arrangement rested on what Mother had told him, so that it would not have been very surprising had he refused to take me on.

The third week I was home, Mother and I made the journey to the hospital to see the new consultant. We went by taxi. On arrival we hung around for hours, whilst I went through all the routine of the Outpatients' department until, at last, I was able to see the surgeon. He was a small, very cheerful man with a lame foot. As I lay there looking at him I began to wonder why he was lame. The thought crossed my mind that perhaps some other doctor had made a bad job of his foot. His attitude was unexpected, for he gave the impression that I was not too seriously ill. He thought it was nothing that an operation would not clear up and added rather casually, he was unable to take me into hospital right then, but would send for me when there was a bed vacant in the ward. (It was much more difficult to get into hospital at that time than it is at present.) Having to return home was something I had not anticipated. I put a good front on it and insisted to Mother that I was well enough to travel by public transport. This we did and both arrived home utterly exhausted, not having eaten for the best part of the day and vaguely worried as to the outcome of this new move.

Mother and myself were greeted by a chorus of questions from the rest of the family, 'What did he say?' I crawled into bed being too tired to talk and Mother gave the report back. My father said he was pleased because it sounded hopeful and set about making some tea for us.

I struggled on at home for over two months. When I finally heard from the hospital I was glad to go, partly because the new specialist had given an optimistic impression and also because I was relieved to be able to give the family a rest. However, my physical condition had deteriorated whilst I was home.

The letter which arrived admitting me into hospital read like a legal document. It bristled with instructions and commands as to what the patient must bring into hospital such as – nightwear, dressing gown, slippers and soap, sugar, butter, eggs and fruit, etc., and what the patient was forbidden, which included alcohol and medicine. The patient was to arrive at a specified time in the morning – neither earlier and certainly not later. Included also were instructions as to the number of visitors allowed, the days and times of visiting and some notes on general behaviour. Finally, the letter was signed with an imposing signature for and on behalf of the Board of Governors. (Despite the saying that comparisons are odious, it is sometimes nice to make them. Many hospitals when admitting patients now include a booklet, the content of which varies slightly. Some give a potted history of the hospital, including pictures. They inform patients not only of what they are supposed to do, but also why. A list of amenities such as ward shopping facilities, hairdressing, mobile telephone service and library, etc. How to recognize the different uniforms amongst the doctors and nurses is also explained, and at least one booklet ends in the hope that the patients will enjoy their stay in hospital!)

Again I made the journey to the hospital by taxi. Although the taxi-driver was kindly and understanding, I found the journey jarring and exhausting. I recall Mother wanting to tip the taxi-driver but he refused any more than the exact fare, saying that he never accepted anything from people going to hospital. It was never suggested I might travel by ambulance: the ambulance service was then very restricted and available only within rigidly defined circumstances.

This new hospital was one of the smaller voluntary hospitals, looking grey and forbidding. I managed to be admitted into the ward with the minimum amount of fuss. The nurse informed me that it was a rule for all new patients to have a bath so, rather unsteadily, I followed the nurse into a small, very untidy bathroom. She helped me undress and said suddenly, 'You don't really need a bath – I'll splash the water about and you slip into bed.' I was more than pleased to comply.

Hospital bathrooms, invariably cluttered with all kinds of gear, were at best untidy, and at worst downright dirty. There never seemed to be enough space with the result that the ward bathroom became a general dumping ground. Neither were the bathrooms designed to provide anything like enough baths or washbasins. This ward in which I had just arrived had eighteen beds, and one small bathroom containing one very deep bath, difficult to get in and out of. The bedpan sluice and lavatories were near the bathroom and not, as in some hospitals, completely separated. This small area contained a miscellany of articles. Included were several large waterproof sheets recently scrubbed, rows of hot-water bottles, wooden blocks for raising the beds, numerous glasses containing urine specimens, numbers of occasionally used gadgets and recently used instruments. In a ward where I was to stay later there were twenty-six beds and one bathroom. It is small wonder that with such conditions the whole time I was in hospital my hair was only washed twice. There was a permanent instruction which went on for years, carried forward from one hospital to the other, to the effect that Nurse will, at some unspecified time in the future, wash my hair. This instruction was handed down from one set of nurses to another and whilst nobody ever forgot, neither did any one carry it out. Having said that, it is only fair to add, so much work not remotely connected with the profession was put upon the nurses, it is small wonder that certain essentials were overlooked. Yet another aspect is that surgical wards did not expect to cater for long-term or chronically sick people.

However, there was this curious dichotomy in the attitude towards cleanliness. On the one hand, all sterilized dressings and treatments were performed with fanatical attention to the smallest detail and on the other hand, was this antiquated Victorian bathroom equipment. Patients unable to get out of bed were supplied with washing bowls twice a day. These bowls were usually large and heavy as they were made from enamel and contained the minimum of water: also, there were occasional blanket baths. On the whole, it can truthfully be said, water was at a premium. Some of those conditions have changed. Hospitals have hairdressers calling at regular intervals and, as a boost to morale, patients are quite rightly encouraged to look civilized. Unfortunately, many of the antediluvian bathrooms still remain as a memorial to the fact that not enough money is provided to build or modernize hospitals.

The ward I was in was not cramped and had a considerable amount of space between each bed. On one side there were three disproportionate mock windows quite small and high up near the ceiling, which added nothing to the light or air of the ward. On the opposite side were the real windows, which looked out on to a courtyard below. Growing in this courtyard was one very large plane tree. From my bed I could see the massive top branches which, from being bare and leafless, I watched spread to full growth. The ward was heated by two combustion stoves and a fireplace. This fireplace at the very end of the ward was small, tiled, with a narrow mantelpiece on the top, of the type that could be found in the parlour of any ordinary house. In the centre of the ward was a huge pillar, into which was built two combustion type stoves. These were all in use. The hospital porter fetched up the coal and the ward maid, as part of her job, used to clean the grates each morning and see that the fires were kept going. A large, oblong table stood in the middle of the ward, with numerous cupboards round the sides, and on the white tiled top stood a china jug and washbasin. This jug and basin were used by the doctors to wash their hands in. During the doctors' round, the nurses were continually backwards and forwards either filling the jug with clean water or emptying and washing the basin. Now there was a small sink on one side of the ward – I never discovered why it was more convenient to use a jug and basin.

It was definitely more cheerful in the previous hospital; this ward was quiet, dreary, with a prison-like effect. One of the reasons may have been the ward door which was huge (it dwarfed the tallest person), very heavy and painted a glaring white. It closed slowly and the effect was claustrophobic, for it seemed to shut the patients into the ward with a finality that created two worlds: the world on the inside of the ward and the world on the other side of the door. I was in this ward over four months and the atmosphere did not affect me at the beginning, though it started to grow on me after the first month. I thought it was just myself that was affected, but others in the ward told me the same thing, that is, they felt not merely shut in but locked in. The atmosphere in hospital wards varies tremendously – it is hard to say why.

Next morning I had the usual visit from the house surgeon who, much to my surprise, was a woman doctor. She was attractive, very feminine and had great charm. Good relations were established after the first visit since I felt very easy with her and she did much afterwards to help tide me over a difficult time. Following her visit was one from the specialist, who greeted me with an expression I was to hear many times. He said, 'And how are you – none the better for my asking?' He was the only consultant I had ever seen who cultivated no bedside manner and was completely devoid of 'side'. He would help himself to anything I happened to have on top of my locker such as sweets or fruit; cut himself buttonholes from flowers in the ward – this with the help of nurses' surgical scissors, then sit on the side of the bed and talk in a perfectly natural way. Between them, the specialist and the house surgeon had the magnetism to put anyone at ease and I certainly did not feel afraid.

After this first visit the specialist had a long talk to Sister away from my bed. Sister afterwards told me that the day of operation had been fixed for the coming Thursday. I was less afraid of this operation than the previous ones, having arrived at the firm conclusion I would have pain and discomfort, but would be able to walk out of the hospital free and well.

Preparation for most major operations was uncomfortable to say the least and this was no exception. It usually started the day before, and the coming event and feeling of pending doom hung over my head like the sword of Damocles.

The day of operation arrived and I just lay and waited. Covered – one could hardly call it dressed – in an enormous grey flannel garment worn back to front, wearing a pair of very thick knitted woollen stockings, my hair covered and tied back from my face, screened off from the rest of the ward patients, the hours dragged by seemingly endless. I had been awake since five o'clock that morning. Nobody uttered a word of explanation. At half past ten there was the usual round of mid-morning drinks for the patients which was served from a trolley. The nurse serving the drinks put her head round the screens and said to me, 'Nothing to drink for you, my dear, you're having an "op" today, aren't you?' 'I'm very thirsty' I told the nurse, but she was adamant – no drink of any description. About an hour later, my tongue felt as though it was cleaving to the roof of my mouth and I looked round for some way to obtain a sip of water. There was always a jug of cold water and a glass left on top of the locker by the side of each patient, though this was carefully omitted in the case of anyone having major surgery of any description, so there was no hope of obtaining a sip of water in that way. At twelve noon the dinners were served, which were brought into the ward one or two at a time, as some of the patients were on diet. Again, the nurse serving dinners pretended I was not there, so I called her and explained how long I had been awake and that I was thirsty. She said, 'When did you last eat?' I told her, I had had a cup of tea and a slice of toast about six o'clock in the morning, that I was definitely not hungry, just very dry. Nurse thought for a moment and said, 'I'll see what Sister says.' She proceeded to serve all the dinners, clear away the plates, do the bed-pan round, help tidy the ward and the beds, whilst I waited patiently for her to return with a drink of water, or at least, a message from Sister. After this, I could hear the change-over of nurses on duty and heard the voice of the staff-nurse, who had returned having had the morning off.

Staff was a very pleasant girl and came round the screen to see how I was faring and give me some moral support. I started once more on the question of the drink which, of course, she knew nothing about, since the previous nurse I had asked and Sister had both gone off duty. Staff Nurse did get me about a quarter of a glass of water, which I drank as though it was nectar. After this I dozed off to sleep for a little while and awoke having no idea of the time, as I was screened off from the wall clock in the ward and did not possess a watch. I tried to guess what the time might be and thought I had been asleep for hours. I called the staff nurse as she passed and asked her the time (it was not yet 2 p.m.). I also asked whether she knew how much longer I would have to wait: she had not the faintest idea. By that time Sister had returned to the ward and four hours later came the first words of explanation: I was told the operation would have to be postponed as the surgeon was unable to come that day. There may have been good reason for the adjournment – I will never know. But to wait from five in the morning until six in the evening and then make such an announcement!

Sister sent in a tray for me with a boiled egg, a pot of tea and bread and butter. I drank all the tea though I could not eat anything, for by that time I had become worked up into a state of acute agitation.

The operation was put off until the following week, after which most of the preparation had to be done again. When I finally went up to the theatre my original feeling of hope and enthusiasm was much dampened by the long wait. I was quiet but churned-up inside and was further dismayed as one of the nurses brought out a long, wide leather strap, which she calmly tied round my legs and firmly buckled up. No action could have been more calculated to increase my fears than being held prisoner by this enormous leather strap. However, all things come to an end and after the usual nightmare of the anaesthetic, I found myself back in the ward.

In the days before the use of electric blankets, there were some primitive arrangements for keeping patients warm and reducing post-operative shock. Aluminium hot-water bottles were widely used which were hard, uncomfortable and dangerously hot for short periods. There were also rubber and stone hot-water bottles though I cannot remember the latter being used in hospital, perhaps because of their weight. For keeping patients warm after operations this hospital used what appeared to be a crude, wire cradle, fitted with rows of electric bulbs. There are, of course, modern versions of this in use at the present time, though the wire cradle to which I refer looked like a real 'do it yourself job'. This was placed over the patient's body with a thin blanket over the top and then switched on. Apparently it served the purpose, though the blaze of light and heat emanating from this contraption was quite frightening.

The result of this operation was absolute disaster. Within hours of it being performed the doctor had to remove the dressing because of the bleeding. There was some talk of my going up to the theatre again, which really reduced me to a state of terror, since I was vomiting badly as a result of the recent anaesthetic. The consultant came back twice to have a look at it and finally decided to leave it alone – to my great relief. About a week later when the sister was changing the dressing I plucked up enough courage to have a look at it and found it hard to believe that part of my body was also part of myself. The specialist, who was much given to puns and banter, kept up a running commentary with the house surgeon, the students and the nursing staff about this piece of surgery; somehow I found it very difficult to join in the fun.

None of the sutures held and there was a gap of some three to four inches between one side of the incision and the other. The house surgeon was very kind to me during this period. She kept reassuring me that Time was a great healer and it would all right itself – perhaps she really believed it. I remember Mother coming to see me about two weeks after this operation. I was in such a state, I almost wanted to ask her to go home, except that it seemed such an awful thing to say. Mother, with her usual intuition, must have divined my thoughts, for she said, 'Perhaps you would like me to go home, so that you can get some sleep.' I did not know what I wanted at the time, except that I was grateful to Mother for going, when she had only just arrived. I do not wish to go any further into the harrowing details, except to say my chances of getting better were almost nil. I became completely bedridden. I did not realize the enormity of what had happened for some time and still thought I would get better, though it might take longer.

The behaviour of doctors and nurses towards the patient always seemed the same – that is, whatever happened to the patient was regarded as normal and in the natural order of things. They discussed treatments and conditions among themselves, but there was a united front towards the patient which might be summed up as, 'this is how it is – it cannot be otherwise'. Logically I suppose this was true. When a thing has happened it has happened. This attitude concealed a great deal from the patient, for it gave the impression that everyone knew exactly what to do and how to meet any unforeseen circumstance. The truth was often the reverse. That most complicated of machines, the human body, is also highly individual. Through long experience certain trends and reactions could be reasonably well gauged, though I came to know through long experience as a patient that doctors were often surprised, sometimes flummoxed and irritated, when things did not work out according to plan. It was this element of surprise and uncertainty that was successfully hidden from the patient. It was (and still is) quite an art.

One day the specialist made a very strange remark. In the course of the usual routine questions and answers he suddenly said to me, 'You must hate me.' I considered this surprising statement and decided there was no one to blame. In taking the decision to bring me to this hospital, Mother had intended only my good and every doctor wants his work to be successful. I have always remembered this conversation, since it was the only time any doctor had ever said a thing like that to me. He was unconventional in the whole of his approach to patients, and I was disconcerted by this remark, especially the use of the word 'hate'. It set me thinking along other lines about the doctor/patient relationship – perhaps it showed me the other side of the coin in a way I had never seen it before.

Sometimes the specialist was amusing. He used to look at the result of this operation and call it 'The Devil's Punchbowl'. He asked me whether I knew where it was and, not having been around very much, I had to confess I did not know. He then asked Nurse if she knew where The Devil's Punchbowl was situated. Nurse, being Irish, insisted that it was in Ireland. Sister came to the rescue and announced it was near Haslemere. I later looked up this question and discovered there were several 'Devil's Punchbowls', including one in Ireland. When I told the nurse the result of my discovery she simply smiled and said, 'I told yer so, me dear.'

In the bed beside mine was an attractive young woman named Kathleen, also recovering from a serious operation and very ill. She was eight years my senior, educated and seemed to me experienced and worldly: neither did those qualities appear incompatible with her religious beliefs, for she was a devout Catholic. She gained a great deal of comfort through her faith and tried hard to imbue me with some of this feeling – I think she succeeded to a certain extent. Kathleen hailed from Southampton of a middle-class family and worked in London as a buyer for a large Kensington store which, in those days before bulk buying, was a responsible and highly paid position. After being in hospital for months following an emergency operation, she went home better. For years afterwards she wrote to me regularly when, quite unexpectedly, I received a letter one day telling me that she had decided to become a nun and was about to enter a Closed Order: she was sending me this letter, her last, with fervent hopes for my ultimate recovery and said she would pray for me every day – which I have no doubt at all she did. This letter was one of the strangest I have ever received. It was calmly written, though its message was irreversible, immutable and final. This happened early in 1932 – I have never heard from her since.

My stay in this hospital dragged from weeks into months. The pain was incessant, though it was somehow more manageable during the day – it was the nights that seemed endless. Sometimes I would fall asleep in the early hours of the morning, only to be awakened by the noise and clatter of washing bowls and bedpans. As patients were neither consulted nor ever given any kind of explanation, it is impossible for me to give an accurate account of the treatment I received. I had something called olive oil infusions, was required to drink medicine which looked like water and tasted so bitter that I retained it with difficulty. I ran a temperature which fluctuated between 103° and 104°, a fact which did not appear to surprise the doctors and they took it as a matter of course. When I stopped taking the medicine my temperature came down – it seemed the high temperature was a side-effect of the medicine. Many years later I was asked by a doctor whether, during the time I had this illness, I had been given arsenic in medicine. Whilst I had to reply I did not know, I have since been of the opinion that there is probably some connection between my retaining traces of arsenic and that medicine. Not forgetting the more glamorous aspects of hospital treatment, at different times I was given brandy and champagne, which did not come with the usual medicine round but was fetched in state, on its own. Some patients in the ward eyed this procedure with some suspicion and could not believe such luxury was part of the treatment. Somehow I did not rise to the occasion that the drinking of champagne seem to warrant, since I have never been able to acquire a palate for drink. I am not teetotal, neither do I think drink is wicked – only stupid in excess. I have never become educated into appreciating the finer points with regard to drink and remain socially unsophisticated in this respect. The general consensus of opinion in the ward was neatly summed up with an economy of words, namely, 'It was a waste to give champagne to me.' I tried to counter this judgment by suggesting that perhaps I was not supposed to enjoy it – after all, it was entered on my treatment card along with all the other concoctions. This was immediately dismissed as sheer heresy. It was forcibly argued that champagne remained champagne and in a class of its own – no matter what.

As a result of this last operation my condition definitely worsened and the future seemed bleak and uncertain.

After four months at this hospital, I noticed a lengthy discussion between the specialist and the ward sister, well away from my bedside. I knew by their glances they were discussing me, though I could not hear a word they said. The specialist used to come into the ward regularly every week: often he did not bother to see me. I started to ask the house surgeon whether she had any idea of what was going to happen. The woman doctor was very kind and always spoke to me as though she had all the time in the world. However, she also had a skilful knack of turning the conversation on to all kinds of other topics and away from its original course, with the result that somehow I never knew any more at the end of the conversation than I knew at the beginning.

There are some people who get to know a great deal of what is going on at any given time, more accurately than numbers of others, whilst themselves playing no part in general organization. All factories have people like that and a considerable amount of information comes the way of caretakers and milkmen. In hospital it was the ward cleaners and orderlies who sometimes knew much more than the patients. They usually knew a good deal about patients, just as much about the staff and were versed in all kinds of titbits of hospital scandal.

The cleaner in this ward had been working in the hospital for years. Her routine did not vary. She lived within walking distance of the hospital and started work at 6.30 a.m. After first doing some jobs in the kitchen, she swept and cleaned the ward in the following way. First, she pulled each bed away from the wall towards the centre of the ward. Her equipment consisted of a large basin of cold tea-leaves, which she sprinkled over the floor to lay the dust before sweeping; a large broom with which she swept up the tea-leaves together with the dust; a bucket of water and a coarse floor flannel. She dipped the flannel into the bucket of water, wrung out the excess water with her hands, folded the flannel over the broomhead in a special way, then proceeded to mop the ward floor a section at a time. Lastly, she pushed each bed back into its original position. Many hospitals now use mechanized equipment for cleaning and polishing, though this still does not apply to all. Fairly recently I was a patient for a short time in one of the old hospitals, which was included in a group headed by the most illustrious name in the country. Every morning a woman cleaned the ward floor in exactly the method I have described, except that she did not use cold tea-leaves.

Like most people who have been in hospital a long time, I knew the ward cleaner well and we used to have a chat most mornings. We started off by discussing the weather, as it was difficult to get a real idea of the temperature outside, because the ward was nearly always overheated. I used to be surprised when some mornings she told me how cold it was and how she did not warm up until she entered the ward. It was during one of these morning conversations that she told me in an undertone, I was going to be moved to another hospital. I was very disturbed by this piece of news and asked where I was going, but there was no more information forthcoming. Since nothing was mentioned during the following week, I thought perhaps this news was not true. However, it turned out to be perfectly accurate.

Some ten days after my conversation with the ward cleaner, the specialist came into the ward and, after gazing thoughtfully at the floor for some time, walked slowly towards my bed. I lay at the far end of the ward, so that unless several beds were screened off, I had an uninterrupted view of what was happening. This was the first time for some weeks he had spoken to me, although he had been in to see his other patients. He was quite straightforward and without any preliminaries he came quickly to the purpose of his visit. He explained to me that the doctor in charge had to satisfy the governors that any patient who occupied a bed for a longer than average period, would either get better or not. I believe he was really saying 'either get better or die', though he did not use the last word. It seemed it was possible to stay in hospital for a long time, if the doctor could satisfy the governors to that end. However, if such an assurance was not forthcoming, the patient must be moved to another hospital where they could keep people for an indefinite period. He bluntly told me that he did not know how long I would take to get better and would therefore have to move to another hospital nearby: Sister would give me all the details. He added he was very sorry, he would like to keep me but he was being pressed by the hospital governors. Consultants hardly ever explained awkward or troublesome situations to the patient concerned – this task was usually given to the house surgeon or sister, so it is only fair to mention that he gave the explanation himself and did not delegate it to someone else. Although I did not know this at the time, he had previously asked to speak to my mother. He told her I had a disease known as actinomycosis and would not live longer than about two years. Mother told me of this conversation years afterwards, when I was better.

Following the conversation about moving to another hospital, which took place in the morning, I had an unexpected visit from Mother in the early afternoon, though it was not formal visiting day. Obviously, she had already been told I was going to be moved and wanted to accompany me to the next hospital. Mother had hardly sat down to speak to me when the ward sister told her the almoner wished to see her – I wondered what she wanted. It seemed this interview was in connection with obtaining an ambulance, since there was no other way in which I could travel. I have already mentioned the restricted use of the ambulance service and one would have supposed the hospital almoner might have used her authority to phone for one. Not at all. Mother was given an address, told whom to contact and on a sultry afternoon during a heatwave, had to walk round an unfamiliar district in order to make the necessary arrangements – not to mention the payment of ten shillings towards the cost. Having made all the arrangements for me to move later in the afternoon, she returned to the hospital exhausted. It was almost two weeks since the ward cleaner had told me what she heard, so the decision had been taken then, yet the actual moving from one hospital to the other was rushed through in little over a day.

I could do little for myself, so Mother packed my few belongings from the locker and we both waited in silence for the ambulance to come. All the ward patients wished me good luck and goodbye. The house surgeon had a chat to me and told me not to worry; she had forwarded all my notes to the new hospital, so that they would know all about me and she would make it her business to find out how I was getting on. At the last minute, one of the nurses who was off-duty rushed in to wish me well. I managed the minimum of polite replies, but seemed unable to sustain any conversation. The journey by ambulance was very short. I had been told the name of the hospital, though it did not mean anything to me and I had no real idea where I was going – in the circumstances perhaps it was as well.

5

ARRIVING by ambulance at this third hospital I could not see the outside of the building, though what I saw of the inside resembled a morgue. The entrance was dark with dingy yellow paintwork: there seemed to be miles of corridors and passageways. It was curiously quiet, having none of the bustle and sense of purpose one usually notices on entering a hospital. There were several old people ambling about who seemed to be dressed in a kind of uniform. I thought it was my imagination they were all dressed alike though I learned afterwards this was not an hallucination and they did, in fact, wear a uniform. I tried to console myself with the thought that perhaps this was the worst side of the building and hoped the ward might not be too bad. This was my first experience of a Poor Law hospital. It was in 1929 and the far-reaching Public Health Act of that year had only just been passed.

I was carried out of the ambulance and transferred on to one of the hospital trolleys which made it easier, as I could be wheeled along instead of carried. With me were the two ambulance men and Mother, holding a small case which contained my belongings. We stopped in front of a large, slow, rickety lift, with heavy outer gates of trellised ironwork, large enough to hold a bed and several persons. We stopped and waited – I wondered why. The lift went up again empty, though when it came down, I noticed it contained a dead body being taken to the mortuary by two porters. Having been in the other two hospitals more than a year I had seen a number of people die, so recognized the covered stretcher arrangement used for that purpose. It seemed ominous that my first encounter in this hospital should be with death. My mother appeared not to have observed the incident and I did not refer to it.

Later, when I was in the ward, I could hear this lift trundling up and down carrying ward deliveries of every description, including food; it served the operating theatre; visitors used it when available and patients who had died were taken to the mortuary in it. If lifts were able to speak, what stories they could tell.

Coming out of the lift which had recently contained the corpse, we had to wait in the corridor outside the ward for two or three minutes. I looked around me. The wards in the other hospitals had always been named, so that I was surprised when I noticed that the ward I was about to enter was merely numbered. When I received letters, following my own name was always the name of the ward. I knew the names perpetuated those who had endowed the ward and the same applied to some of the beds. I always suffered as much from loss of freedom through being in hospital as from any other cause, so that the number had a strange effect on me: in a curious way, it made me feel like someone whose identity as an individual had been destroyed.

As I was wheeled through the door I was astounded by the size of the ward – it was simply enormous. It was not only long but exceptionally wide. There were four rows of beds very close together, with only just enough room between each row to move around. At one end of the ward was a long row of cot-beds with the adjustable sides drawn up. These cot-beds had frightening associations with old-age, senility and incontinence, where life had turned full cycle and people returned to their childhood. There was also a strange noise which seemed to be coming from outside the ward. I could not place this at first, though I later traced it to the clanking noise of the trams. This ward faced a main road, where the sounds of the trams jangling unevenly along the lines, stopped only for a few hours when it was very late.

I was put into a bed along one of the inner rows, far away from the light of any of the windows. My spirits sank and I felt overwhelmed as I looked round this sea of beds and faces. (The entire concept of sick people being laid out in rows has always appalled me, yet most hospitals still retain this pattern.)

The nurse came over, looked at me and my belongings and told Mother to take my nightdress home. She said that the hospital supplied nightwear and did not allow patients to wear their own clothes. I took off my thin nightie, gave it to Mother and I was given the hospital nightgown. This garment, made from coarse, grey flannelette, was so hard and stiff I did not have the strength to unfold it and Mother helped me to get into it. The weather was very hot, and on this summer's day I was enveloped in this monstrous garment, which dragged a full half yard over my legs, with wide, gathered sleeves almost twice as long as my arms – I felt I could scarcely breathe because of the weight. It is difficult to imagine such a scene in the twentieth century; it was more in keeping with 1829 than 1929.

Mother stayed a while longer. I could tell she was also upset by those stupid, needless regulations, though she tried to make light of it by saying, 'anyway, everyone is treated alike, so there is no favouritism'. Mother lingered on for as long as she was able and was finally asked to go home. For the first time, my entire reserve broke down and I could not stop weeping. Nurse came up and assured me in a matter of fact way, 'Everyone feels the same when they first arrive, you will get used to it in time.'

Looking back over this period I am better able to place it in perspective. The two previous hospitals I had been in were voluntary. I now found myself in a Poor Law hospital attached to the workhouse. This explained the rules with regard to clothing and why people appeared so odd when I first saw them – they were, in fact, dressed in the workhouse regulation clothes. I was in an institution which belonged more to the London of Charles Dickens than the beginning of the nineteen-thirties. For example, the workhouse master and matron had only recently relinquished their posts. These posts were administrative and they were directly responsible to the guardians. The attitude towards people in this hospital was one of the treatment of paupers, which was still retained as it had been for the last hundred years. As I have already said, the Law which empowered the London County Council to take over and administer the workhouses had only just been passed. The changeover took years to have full effect and I came into this hospital before any perceptible change had taken place.

One of the arrangements made during this time was that voluntary hospitals could, by mutual consent, get rid of their long stay and chronic sick patients by sending them to the newly constituted council hospitals. It was obviously pressure of this nature that obliged the specialist to have me moved here. Two and a half years later I was in a voluntary hospital where the sister would threaten to transfer any patient, whom she considered difficult or unco-operative to a nearby Council hospital. However, I have jumped ahead and must return to my story.

This hospital consisted of several very large wards. There was no Outpatients' department and, so far as I could see, few amenities in the way of specialized treatment other than an operating theatre. The ward in which I now found myself was mainly geriatric. Some patients were there due to accidents and in this connection I remember a young woman with a broken leg. She was in a state of perpetual indignation, not so much because of the fracture as because she had been run over by an ambulance: she regarded this combination of circumstances as a conspiracy. Opposite me was a young girl aged thirteen who had been ill a matter of years. There might have been other young chronic sick though I did not know many patients on the farther side, because the ward was so large.

The nursing staff were of a different background and educational level than those in the voluntary hospitals, though they were certainly not unkind and did their best in antiquated buildings with outmoded, limited equipment. There was one doctor for the entire ward, a man in his early thirties, uncommunicative and tired-looking, which was not surprising as he always seemed to be on duty. I almost expected him to be on duty for ever and was mildly surprised to see another doctor on night duty. Although the ward doctor was taciturn, he was also very conscientious. As I came to know him better, I decided that having to be responsible for this enormous ward, he was faced with an impossible situation. He was also very different outside his ward duties, according to what my parents told me about him.

At various intervals my parents would arrange a meeting with the ward doctor in the hope he might be able to throw fresh light on my illness. If my father was well enough and the interview with the doctor could be arranged at a time so that my father could attend, both my parents would speak to him. However, most times Mother used to do this on her own, as these interviews were either on week days, or the weather might be bad, in which case my father would be unable to accompany Mother. It so happened that both my parents were able to come to see the ward doctor at this hospital. In view of the doctor's attitude on the ward, where he was very much a man of few words, I was surprised when my parents told me how interested and friendly he was. So far as I could make out the ward doctor asked my parents many more questions about me than vice versa. My father told me that he commented on the fact it was very rare to see such an appendix complication in a hitherto healthy young person like myself. Although the doctor was unable to give any more definite information than was already known about me, he seemed to reassure my parents that I had many advantages on my side such as youth, previous good constitution and so far as he could see, no active sign of malignant disease. This last observation was in direct contradiction to what the previous specialist had said. The manner in which doctors talk to patients' relatives can be very important, for although the ward doctor did not know what was likely to happen to me, he did succeed in giving my father and mother a more hopeful outlook. My father said the doctor spoke to himself and Mother for quite a time and did not seem at all hurried. I remember this doctor well – his name was Dr Izzard.

I have never, before or since, been in a hospital ward where so many people died. Almost every night someone died and occasionally there were as many as four deaths. Of course, not everyone died during the night. Even if people died in the daytime, other ward patients might not know, as the body would not be taken out of the ward until late evening, often many hours after death. We were sure in the morning, because the bed would be freshly made up and empty. All this was not as sinister as it sounds. Then, as now, the problem of the aged sick was a very difficult one. Not to have to die in the workhouse was the unspoken prayer and greatest wish of many aged, working-class people. The family of the aged did their best, often in the face of unemployment and great poverty. Having nursed an aged person for a long time, the difficulties towards the end became more than the ordinary family could cope with, so it was that many of these old folk were finally brought into hospital, literally dying. Sometimes they would last a few weeks, whilst others died overnight. It was this which largely accounted for the death rate and also for the incessant noise.

If my first impression of this hospital was one of quiet this must have been a daytime illusion, for the noise in the ward at night beggared description. Due to the size of the ward it was almost impossible to keep it quiet. Added to this was not only the problem of the aged, but also the number of infirm and hopeless patients unable to do anything for themselves without help. To give just one example. Mrs Livermore was a middle-aged woman, bedridden for years, so crippled with arthritis that all she could move were her eyes. I clearly recall her face with a high, florid colour and all her joints completely locked. To change her position, it took two nurses for she had to be lifted bodily, and also fed. There were a great number of patients suffering from varying degrees of paralysis and many complicated surgical cases, such as my own. All this, in addition to the ordinary noise level: the truth was this ward was unmanageable.

Speaking of noise it was, and still is, a permanent, almost insuperable difficulty. Some of the reasons for noise were intriguing. The night nurses would come on duty feeling active and energetic. They would enter the ward with the lights already dimmed and everyone spoke in whispers. By normal standards of time it was certainly not late – it was just that night time in this hospital began in the late afternoon. There was little convenience for anyone, with the result that the nurses walked miles in and out and to and fro, in this large ward. Neither could this be avoided during the night. The words the night nurse repeated most often were, 'Shss, why don't you go to sleep?' There was always somebody wanting something, not least being the clatter of bed pans. A considerable amount of treatment was given at night, which the nurses were expected to do, taking care to perform every action in a muted kind of way; this was virtually impossible, especially as the night nurse did a great deal of work with the aid of a pocket torch. The patients used to insist that some nurses were born clumsy and as a result of this phenomenon, created more noise at night. Every sound was magnified and seemed to echo. It was rather hard on those high-spirited nurses to have to conform to this artificial pattern of enforced silence. The patients were sometimes fractious and unreasonable; loud complaints would be heard during the night with the inevitable reply of the night nurse, 'Shsss, you're keeping the ward awake.' In cases of acute illness or death, everything went by the board. The lights were full on, there was coming and going by the doctor, the nurses, the night sister and the patients' relatives. The high death rate accentuated the perpetual problem of noise in this ward. For most part the night nurses took all this in their stride – it was part of the job. They used to do much longer periods on night duty, as the schedule was then organized on a basis of three months on nights, alternating with three months on day duty. It was small wonder that the nurses sometimes became irritable towards the end of the night duty period – the strain was really too much.

Having been unable to sleep for most of the first night I arrived at this hospital, partly because I was upset by the rules and regulations and mainly because of the noise, I dozed off in the morning, only to be awakened very sharply by a sudden jerking movement of my bed.

Sisters vary in the manner in which they run the ward. Some sisters concentrate on the organizational side and do little practical work. Others do as much work as the nurses; and I have been in wards where the sister tried to do the work almost single handed – especially when the nurses' off-duty time created brief periods of acute staff shortage. The sister on this ward was young, tall, attractive and very well groomed. One could see that she took great pride in her appearance. This may also have reflected itself in her attitude towards the general appearance of the ward, since she had what amounted to a phobia about the angle and position of the beds. Each morning with unfailing regularity she stood at the entrance of the ward and gave directions, as two of the nurses pushed every bed into the precise position required. Sister maintained a running commentary to the nurses, instructing them as to the number of inches back and forth, or to the right or left, she desired the beds to be pushed. A minor mathematical crisis arose at the points where the beds angled, in order to form a horseshoe shape. This time-consuming exercise took best part of an hour, as there were a large number of beds; when sister was off-duty, the nurse in charge did this as part of her normal ward work. As every bed contained a patient it was difficult to move the bed without the patient knowing. So it was that the sudden jerking of my bed woke me up on that first morning.

The next thing to amaze me in this hospital was the food; both the quality of the food and the way in which it was cooked and served. There was actually more food in this Poor Law hospital, though of such poor quality and so badly cooked, most of it was uneatable. However, it was the way in which the ward tea was served that never ceased to be both fascinating and revolting. The tea, with soda added to make it stronger, arrived in a large, discoloured urn and was poured from a tap on the side. The milk was already made with the tea, so we had to drink it as it came. It came looking like brown ale and tasted like a brew made from bitter herbs.

The cups, plates and other utensils were so weighty, most of us did not have the strength to hold them. There were very few bed-tables, so that most food and drink had to be balanced on the very small space on top of the locker. Many a time I noticed the more feeble patients left their food and drink, simply because they were unable to manage it properly, since the nurses never had enough time to look after all those who needed help.

The food situation at that time was bad in most hospitals. In both the voluntary hospitals I was in before coming here, the food was so poor in quality and little in quantity, that it was impossible to be reasonably fed without the patients' friends or family bringing food into the hospital. For example, in theory if the patients did not have an egg, the kitchen should have supplied one: in practice, if the patient did not have an egg, he went without. Sick people are usually finnicky about food, but there was no choice – one accepted what was given or went without.

All hospitals had to cater for special diets and some of us wished we could be included, because they had food which we on ordinary diet never tasted. There were slight variations between different hospitals with regard to food. Ordinary diet was roughly as follows. At 6 a.m. there was an early morning cup of tea, though in this Poor Law hospital the early morning tea urn arrived from the main kitchen, as there were very few patients well enough to be able to make tea for this huge ward. Breakfast at 8 a.m. consisted of porridge, tea, two half slices of bread, rather stale as it had been cut hours before, and an egg, if available. Each morning as the nurse collected the eggs from patients, she would mark them in pencil with the number of the bed. The eggs when boiled were either forgotten and emerged as hard as bricks, or the time underestimated and they were runny. As the nurse who boiled the eggs did this alongside several other jobs, occasionally the eggs were boiled all right but remained in the kitchen temporarily forgotten and, when they were hurriedly remembered, were distributed cold when breakfast was nearly finished. Sometimes bacon was served for breakfast, though never with an egg. There were also surprise items. I remember a very young nurse moving swiftly round the ward asking whether anybody wanted fish for breakfast. If the answer was 'yes', two undersized sardines appeared on a large plate. Mid-morning there was a drink served, usually Ovaltine, milk or coffee and oddly enough, in one hospital, milky rice pudding. Very few of the patients drank the coffee, since it was made from strange-tasting coffee essence and had a dubious flavour. Lunch at twelve noon consisted of meat, vegetable, under-cooked potatoes and I especially recall all this swimming in a thin, watery gravy. The sweet was mostly semolina or rice. There was a limited amount of chicken for people who were very ill and a great deal of thought was given by Sister as to who should partake of this delicacy. For afternoon tea at three o'clock there was bread and butter and jam with the tea and a small cake on Sundays. There was sometimes fish for the evening meal though more often the eternal mincemeat, followed by a drink – this was at 6.30 p.m. Set out in this way the day's food sounds adequate but so much of it was not eaten. Because the food was monotonous and unappetizing there was enormous waste at all meals. It was regularly said in the ward at mealtimes that the nurse took out more than she brought in. There was little decent food though we had a great deal of medicine which, we were told, was good for us.

From the early evening meal it was a long time to go until next morning, so that there was a good deal of surreptitious eating during the night – especially after visiting days when stocks of food were highest. It depended who was on duty at night for sometimes as a favour, nurse would make a cup of tea for the patients.

Apparently food for nurses was not much better, for they complained about it in every hospital I was in and would accept food, fruit or sweets from the patients. Oddly enough, people in hospital think and talk a great deal about food, even if they are unable to eat very much. They would wistfully mention all manner of choice dishes they would eat in large quantities, if only it was available. Such conversation often passed the time of day.

It was the general attitude towards food that was so strange. There were no heated trolleys at that time, so the nurses carried the plates of food into the ward from the adjoining kitchen and because of the vast amount of work they had to get through, there was no time for civilized eating. Meals were regarded as a necessary evil, to be surmounted as quickly as possible so that, from start to finish, speed was the watchword.

I spent several Christmases in hospital. The miracle of the improved cooking for Christmas and Boxing Day was always a source of wonder in the ward. The meals were delicious. So far as we knew, there was the same cook in the same kitchen and whilst the Christmas food was of higher quality and more plentiful, it was the standard of cooking that was so much better. Alas, after Boxing Day we reverted to the standard of food previously described, until the following Christmas.

Time dragged in this ward. As usual, there was nothing to do. The only break in the deadly monotony were the two visiting periods, Wednesday and Sunday. By this time, I had developed a large area of extreme soreness round the wound which most doctors who had not seen it before, thought was a burn. One day I said to the doctor, 'That part of me looks like a skinned rabbit.' The doctor laughed – he must have thought this description of myself neither scientific nor poetic. This wound gave me years of pain and made it difficult for me to concentrate, though I did try to read every day. I was almost completely cut off from friends I had known at home, although some wrote or very occasionally paid me a visit. This ward was particularly lonely because of the number of helpess and aged people. There are many forms of loneliness, though one of the worst is that of being surrounded by people day and night and never being able to get away. This may sound like a contradiction in terms, but, in a ward full of people, the sense of being trapped and isolated became really acute. In some ways it was like being in a prisoner-of-war or other type of camp, where human beings were forced to live in close proximity and could not get away either from each other or from the place where they were being held. This crushing and debilitating feeling rendered people almost powerless and it was very common among the chronic sick. The feeling was spasmodic and eventually passed though, while it passed, the cycle of time seemed not merely to slow down, but grind to a halt.

Some of the patients occupied themselves with knitting or sewing that their visitors brought into the ward. One of the most industrious was a lady named Miss Martin, who was in the next bed to mine. She was simply enormous and had been in bed for years. She was a relatively young woman with quite pleasing features, though it seemed difficult to determine her age. She was a Scot and I do not know how or why she was in this hospital. She kept herself very busy and did a lot of knitting and crochet work. One day when she was working on a very pretty pattern, I asked her how she did it. But Miss Martin had a great deal of craft prejudice and was not prepared to divulge any information about what she was doing or how she did it. Nothing might have happened about this chance question, except that one of the nurses heard me ask it. Nurse took this refusal up with Miss Martin, who explained that Scottish patterns were traditional and secret. This explanation exasperated Nurse even more and she reported the matter to Sister. The ward sister was rather in the position of the ship's captain and had the final word in all ward disputes. She took the matter quite seriously and remonstrated with Miss Martin, notwithstanding that I said the matter was not important to me. Sister made a moral issue of this, pointing out all patients in hospital carried a burden and that her attitude was not in the right spirit. Sister ended this homily by almost ordering her to show me how to crochet the pattern. Miss Martin obeyed the instruction and showed me how to do it: while so doing, she assured me she bore me no ill will over this affair and was in reality very pleased that I was now fortunate enough to be initiated into the secret art of Scottish patterns.

I was unable to concentrate much on handwork of any description, so the argument that took place over the crochet pattern was hardly worth the effort. It seemed as though nothing whatever was happening. I had no treatment other than dressings, not that this is intended as a criticism against the hospital, for in the past I had had a great deal done, with results hardly spectacular. In this connection I am reminded of a quotation I read recently, 'The art of being a good doctor often depends on knowing when to do nothing.'

The ward doctor did the round each morning, with a special round on Fridays, when he examined all the patients in the ward: this took hours there were so many of us, and to finish the round, he often returned after lunch. On one such Friday the doctor said, 'How did you manage to get into this state?' I was confronted by those unanswerable questions from time to time and was always taken aback. Perhaps the doctor was thinking out loud or just being chatty and I tended to jump the gun. After all, he could not say I would get better next week or next month and be able to go home. I was edgy and read into the question certain implications and overtones that the responsibility was entirely mine. I thought, true, I went to see the previous specialist of my own free will and consented to the operation. Continuing this train of thought I felt bitterly, had the operation been a success, no doubt the surgeon would have been the greatest; since it was a failure, for which I did not blame him, I nevertheless resented the idea that I was to blame.

The surgeon who performed this last operation came to see me several times. He used to suddenly appear at irregular intervals. It was very hard to hold anything against him for he exuded goodwill and a feeling of bonhomie. As usual he kept up a running conversation on disconnected subjects ranging from surgery to sport. I often wondered why he came since he had no connection at all with this Poor Law hospital. Perhaps I was on his conscience, or he was trying to work out what went wrong at that last operation. One of the patients wrote and told me that he came and asked to see me when I had already been moved to another hospital.

I continued to lie in bed and became progressively less able to move. For months I had experienced difficulty when trying to sit up in bed and one day I noticed with a shock that both my legs were so stiff that I was only able to bend them with great effort. Even simple exercises might have saved me some of the misery I endured later, as a result of not being helped to move about more, although this difficulty of movement cetainly did not start in this hospital. I went on this way for several months, when a change in my circumstances came about through totally unexpected outside forces.

One Wednesday afternoon Mother came to see me as usual and told me of a visit she received from an official connected with the local health authority in the district in which I lived – some seven miles away. As was Mother's habit, she first described the man's appearance – he was tall, well spoken and businesslike. She then came to the more important part, which was the purpose of his visit. It seemed that my being in a hospital outside my own area had created an administrative problem. The charge for my upkeep was the responsibility of the local authority where I lived and that they had to send this money to the present hospital. It was therefore suggested it would be easier for all concerned if I were moved to my own area. Mother was urged to go and visit the local council hospital and was assured she would find it altogether better and more modern. The far-reaching Poor Law Act of 1929 was beginning to operate.

I have already made several references to the change in administration of the Poor Law hospitals which took place at this period. The passing of this new Act gave rise to a tremendous amount of infighting between the various factions concerned. The government of the time, responsible for implementing this Act, were afraid of giving too much power to the local authorities, since such action might disconcert the British Medical Association. The BMA naturally kept a watchful eye on the proceedings. There was considerable difference of opinion between the doctors themselves, some of whom were sympathetic, though many were afraid that the Act would eventually make all doctors civil servants and thus end private practice. There was also sharp discussion about the status of nurses. The standard of entry for voluntary hospital nurses started at a fairly high level: all the nurses I remember had matriculated from grammar or private schools. The newly formed council hospitals were faced with a multitude of problems, not least being the massive reorganization necessary to train many more nurses. Conditions of employment in council hospitals was slightly better – the hours of work were shorter and the pay a little higher. Working as they did on the two-shift system, the hours of work for all nurses were fantastically long. As late as 1936 the hours of duty for nurses were fixed at fifty-four hours a week.

The basic law of 1929, making local authorities responsible for the Poor Law hospitals, was compulsory legislation. Within this framework, however, a great deal of permissive legislation was possible, so that there were differences between the various local authorities and some were much more progressive than others. It was against this background that my mother, on the advice she had been given, decided to visit the council hospital in the area in which I lived. She was very favourably impressed and reported back to me that it looked altogether a better and more modern place. Mother advised me to go there.

My first reaction was that I did not see much point in changing hospitals again, for no better reason than to make it easier for administrative purposes. Although I was very unhappy here, I had suddenly become tired of moving from one hospital to another. At a low ebb, I had arrived at the stage where it did not matter to me very much where I stayed. I was surprised at the change in myself. When I first came here the most important thing seemed how I could get out. Apart from a miracle, it was unlikely that I would suddenly get better. I used to spend hours trying to think out a feasible plan of escape, yet, when the possibility arose, I showed little enthusiasm. After months in this hospital I hardly knew most of the other patients. It was a restless, noisy ward, ill lit and crammed with beds though, worst of all, was the atmosphere of utter dejection. One side of the ward did have a long row of large windows. I was well away from these windows on the opposite side with virtually nothing to look at, except dozens of black, iron beds, for most part occupied by aged and hopelessly ill people. This scene did not vary from the day I arrived until the day I left.

Mother used all her powers of persuasion, which were considerable, to induce me to go and I was finally won over. After five months at this present hospital I was moved, again by ambulance, to the one in my own area.

6

THE separation of the sick from the paupers can be traced to the nineteenth century and has an interesting history.

Workhouses were opened in the first place for paupers and not intended to house the sick. The definition of a pauper was very specifically laid down to mean a person lower in status than the poorest worker or agricultural labourer. The classification of a pauper was almost like that of a criminal. The harsh way in which workhouses were controlled, was meant to demonstrate to society that those dregs of humanity who entered there were certainly not going to be pampered. From this attitude followed the policy of the boards of guardians, who were responsible for their administration. The word 'pauper' included almost every age group from mothers with babies to the destitute aged. Also included were the sick, the insane and mental defectives. The organization was not intended to raise the level of the inmates, but to prevent those above the accepted definition from entering the workhouse. Yet few things are wholly bad, for in this severe, rigorous, uncompromising way it did provide a roof over the heads of the otherwise destitute homeless, together with a place to sleep and sufficient food to keep alive.

Originally workhouses made no proper provision for the treatment of the sick paupers though, during the nineteenth century, the government was forced to take action because of the spread of infectious diseases. As a result isolation hospitals were extended and rebuilt: from this began a network of hospitals attached to the workhouse for the treatment of general illness. As recently as 1965, when it was demolished, one of those truly dreadful old workhouses was sited facing Baker Street station in London. It was known as Luxborough Lodge, though it was, in fact, the old St Marylebone workhouse, whose origin went back to the eighteenth century. The name was changed in 1948 when the National Assistance Act was introduced.

The history of this place makes interesting if terrifying reading in *The St Marylebone Workhouse and Institute 1730–1965* by. A. R. Neate. Originally the inmates worked twelve to fourteen hours a day under a taskmaster, whose name and image was later changed to a supervisor. Different types of work for able-bodied paupers included spinning and winding yarns, carpentry, tailoring, nursing and domestic work, etc. For those who did not conform to the workhouse rules, there was picking oakum. There were, of course, the workhouse master and matron. Punishments for misbehaviour or running away included flogging for both sexes and starvation diet with hard labour. The first inmates of the St Marylebone workhouse were unmarried mothers and their babies, the majority of whom had been domestic servants. One of the records includes how an infant was left at the workhouse door with the following verse pinned to her clothing:

I am little Kitty, my parents are poor,
I crave your pity, now I am left at your door,
I do not despair but hope I do cherish
I shall be taken care of, as I am left to the Parish.

I often passed this workhouse right up to 1965 when it was demolished. For some time I did not know the origin of this building though, when I discovered the truth, I looked at the old people with different eyes. In warm weather they used to sit outside on wooden benches or walk in the grounds of this large, dreary place. Part of the grounds faced the main road. It was astonishing to observe this workhouse, a relic of a bygone age, facing a modern main road near some of the most expensive property in London. The old people were often wrapped in grey and red blankets, and many of them looked as though death would come as a friend and an ally. I had never seen the inside of this place and was not surprised when a friend of mine, an observant and highly intelligent young woman, burst into tears when describing to me a visit she had made to someone inside this old people's home. She said, and I quote her words, 'There was not an easy chair for the old people to sit on, or an atom of comfort in the entire place.' It was a living reminder of what it means to be old and destitute.

As attitudes towards poverty and illness became more humane, and though overall policy by successive governments included certain improvements, there was no major change until the Act of 1929–30. As I have already said, part of this Act depended on permissive legislation. Within the existing framework there were considerable differences between individual local authorities as to how this law was implemented. Hence, the enormous difference between the hospital I had just arrived at and the one I had left.

The ex-Poor Law hospital in my own area where I arrived towards the end of 1929, was definitely better. From the outside all these hospitals looked alike. A succession of long, rather narrow, five-storey grey buildings, known as blocks. These blocks, named in alphabetical order, were connected by draughty passageways, covered overhead but open on either side, of the type sometimes found linking warehouses together. They were all built around the same time, for I can call to mind five of these hospitals in London, still much in use at the present time, all built on the same principle. Many have since been improved, the open passageways covered in and made part of the main structure, though when I arrived there, no building alterations were being thought of. There was a Casualty room but no proper Outpatients' department. When I arrived by ambulance I was taken into a receiving room, which adjoined the porter's lodge, just inside the main gates. There were in fact two sets of main gates; one leading into the hospital and the other, on a side street, which was the entrance to the workhouse.

I was put into a ground floor ward which contained twenty-six beds. True, the beds were so close together that by leaning over the patients could quite easily touch, yet the ward itself was brighter, cleaner and much more cheerful than the ward in the previous hospital.

There was certainly no cheering by a reception committee to announce my arrival. The ward was full of fracture and surgical cases needing dressing and treatment. I mention fractures because certain types were almost hopeless at that time. The ward sister eyed me with a grim expression when looking through my case history. Turning to the staff nurse she said, 'Fancy sending me this, as though the ward is not heavy enough already!' Unable to walk, with a nasty wound, I had to gloomily admit to myself that I was a lot of extra work. However, I thought it rather unfair of Sister to expect the patients' illnesses to conform to specification so as to fit the needs of the ward.

I arrived at the hospital in the morning, in time to see the doctor on the routine ward round. As in the other hospital there was one doctor with just as much work to do, since he was in charge of other wards besides. The doctor was a young man under thirty, very tall and big built, with an expansive, jolly attitude towards the patients, the staff and life in general. He entered the ward like Rhadames returning from battle in the first act of *Aïda*. Sister obviously enjoyed doing the round with him, and pointed out I was a new arrival from another hospital. The doctor asked me how long I had been ill (it was almost two years), how long since my last operation and then said to Sister, 'Put her next to Milly, they will be able to compare notes.' I wondered who Milly was and what we had in common. To find out I did not have long to wait.

After the midday meal, my bed and belongings were moved to the far end of the ward next to a very attractive redhead, who was obviously Milly. She turned to me with a very cheerful 'hullo', and asked where I came from. She looked a very petite girl, red haired and freckled, with a very cheerful grin: nobody looked less like an invalid than Milly. Continuing the conversation, she asked in a forthright way, 'What's the matter with you?' I replied rather vaguely, 'Oh, it's a complicated story.' She assured me that so was her story and proceeded to tell me something of herself, as she remarked, 'To get it over with.' Hers was really quite an extraordinary story.

Milly told me she was twenty-four years old – a few years older than myself, though she neither looked her age nor older than me. Engaged to be married, she had suddenly started an attack of acute appendicitis and, like myself, matters had complicated. She had been in a voluntary hospital for eighteen months and in the present hospital nearly three years. She was unable to remember exactly how many operations she had but, thought it to be in the region of fifteen. So began an association with Milly which ended with her death at the age of forty, having been ill over twenty years – more than half her life. I have never met anybody who behaved less like an invalid than Milly. I then told her something of myself and found we certainly had things in common.

My gaze then passed to Milly's bed and the surrounding area. It was an extraordinary sight. It was hung round with drawstring bags of many shapes and colours; similar bags also adorned her locker. Every available space on the windowsill behind her bed was used for tins, packages and bundles of varying sizes. I was secretly astonished that the ward sister allowed all this but, Milly had a way with her, as I learned as time went by. Displayed in a prominent position on her bedtable was the following notice in large, clear handwriting. 'WHILE I AM VERY PLEASED TO TALK TO ANYBODY WHO WISHES TO CONVERSE WITH ME, I AM NOT PREPARED TO DISCUSS OPERATIONS, SYMPTOMS OR ILLNESS OF ANY DESCRIPTION.'

Most patients in hospital love to discuss themselves and would describe their illnesses to anybody willing to listen. This is understandable since nothing is so important to the person concerned than a breakdown of the body functions. Milly, having been in the ward for years, had heard all this before *ad nauseam* and was determined not to allow a conversation of this nature to get off the ground. She had a great deal to contend with physically, yet she retained a drive and vitality quite remarkable for a girl hopelessly ill. Perhaps the best way to illustrate this would be to describe a day in her life at the hospital.

Except at certain times when Milly really had a setback, she slept fairly well. She would be wide awake as early as four in the morning, nag the night nurse to bring her a washing bowl, would proceed to wash and then spend a long time doing her hair. Milly had the most beautiful copper-coloured hair. She first wetted her hair then very deftly curled it round her fingers, and finally tied the mass of curls back with a ribbon. By that time the early morning tea was brought round and I noted with satisfaction that the tea was made in a teapot and not in an urn. Milly did not bother much with tea and rarely finished the cupful. With her ablutions and hair-do completed, she really started the day's work – the reason for all the parcels and bags then became clear. She made elaborate pincushions and sold them by the score – especially near Christmastime. The pincushions consisted of a silk bag filled with sand, which she then covered with hand-crocheted lace. In the centre of the cushion sat a celluloid doll, clad in a crochet dress. The pincushions were made in a two-colour scheme and, though quite complicated, it was surprising how quickly she made them up. Milly worked at these solidly for most of the day, stopping for meals and dressing, etc. Occasionally Sister became rather cross, suggested she put away her work and give herself a rest: this she did, rather grudgingly. Time was money.

In the days when work therapy was unknown in hospitals, when nothing was done to try and prevent chronic sick patients from becoming seriously depressed, Milly had organized her own system. Moreover, she made quite a few shillings each week selling her pincushions to other patients and their visitors. Every visiting time there were a stream of callers slipping across to Milly's bed to negotiate small matters concerning orders and payment. Speaking of money, she received the princely sum of four shillings a week as a permanent disablement benefit. The amount paid was not uniform and some people received more.

Whilst Milly did most of the work herself, she had no hesitation in trying to enlist the help of any willing person. She drove her family frantic with the list of materials she required, all of which had to be brought into the hospital from the outside. I think that Milly was somewhat disappointed in me, for she hinted one day she had envisaged me as a potential partner in the work scheme and what a wonderful idea it would be for us to work together. Unfortunately there were two serious disadvantages. Firstly, that I was unable to sit up for long periods and secondly, I had neither the energy nor the patience to co-operate with such a project; so that quite early in our association I was written off as a dead loss so far as work was concerned.

Of all the people I met over the years I was in hospital, no one is so engraved in my memory as Milly. Beset as she was with a disability and serious difficulties, having to spend her life in the highly charged, abnormal conditions of hospitals, she was able to cut across all this and manage to create for herself a semblance of rationality and normal life.

I cheered up considerably here, because I was on a ground floor ward and able to look out of the window. I could see people walking to and fro. I suffered less from the awful feeling of claustrophobia, caused through being incarcerated in a huge ward, high up, with almost no human contact apart from the staff and other patients. Looking out of this window made me feel closer to the outside world. I used to watch visitors coming and going, as well as the nurses during their various duty changes. Something was always happening in the grounds outside the ward. Looking out of the window had another curious effect on me – I began to transpose myself and believe it was me walking outside. This impression became so powerful, I was able to use it as an imaginary escape route. To the present day I am able to capture the feeling of make-believe that I was outside and not inside the ward, more distinctly than the day of my actual homecoming.

Facing this ward was another, separated by the corridor. Although these two wards had different numbers they were treated as one, with the same sister and doctor in charge. The doctor always started his morning round opposite, then crossed over and continued in this ward. The doctor's round was always something of an event, as all kinds of important decisions were taken. On my second morning here the doctor said to Sister, 'I am going to get Violet out of bed and walking if it's the last thing I do – I really think she could go home.' The doctor, being a big man with a booming voice, could easily be heard; Sister gave him her special smile of agreement. (The ward sister never argued with the doctor, even if she privately thought him dead wrong.) That morning the doctor spent a long time with me, making various suggestions to Sister concerning treatment. One of his suggestions was to try white of egg as a dressing. When the dressing came to be done, there was the rather strange spectacle of the nurse breaking an egg and trying to separate the white from the yoke. This line of treatment was very short-lived, because if anything it made matters worse; as the egg white was very astringent the pain became unbearable.

Having heard the name 'Violet' mentioned, I asked Milly who

she was. Milly told me that she was a young woman from the ward opposite who had been in hospital longer than herself. She had suspected TB and needed a certain amount of attention. I was rather puzzled about all this since rules for being in or out of bed were rigidly enforced. If one did not feel well at home it was possible to lie down, but not in hospital. Being up meant just that, and if a patient had a relapse they went back to bed again and stayed there. Such was the either/or attitude. Patients were allowed up for short periods soon after operations but this stage did not last long. So how did it come about that Violet was able to get up and did not? And might even have been able to go home!

A week later Violet walked into this ward rather unsteadily and spoke to Milly; obviously the doctor had got her up out of bed. She was a tall, very thin girl in the early twenties and stooped like an old person. Milly introduced me and I used to talk to her. I was surprised to learn that she lived right out of the area, over the other side of London, near Fulham. It seemed her mother was a widow who went out to work and there would be no one to look after her if she went home. Violet really did seem ill, though there was considerable doubt as to how ill she was. Some three weeks later she disappeared – whether home, or to a hospital in her own area I do not know. Possibly she was moved for the same reason as myself, since she was outside the area in which she lived. This was never made clear.

Violet might have been quite ill. A good deal was known about pulmonary TB at that time, though other forms of this disease were not always easy to establish. I thought about it from another angle. Would it be possible for a person in hospital a long time to opt out of normal life? I could understand this attitude in the aged, but for a young woman in her twenties – it seemed to go against nature. The doctor was very firm in his approach, so he must have been satisfied she was not actively tubercular as this hospital had a special ward for that complaint. (I was told by a girl who had been in the TB ward, that it was full of young people.)

I used to think about Violet and wonder how she was getting along. This incident seems to bring into question the entire system of treatment in Poor Law and the early council hospitals.

The ward doctor was in absolute and complete control. With

the exception of certain week-ends, night duty and holiday periods, we rarely saw another doctor in the ward. He may have been answerable to the medical superintendent, about whom I shall have more to say later; so far as the patients knew, he took all the decisions. At best this relationship is weighted against the patient, since he or she is not in possession of specialized knowledge and has to accept all information on trust. That medicine is not an exact science has long been recognized and the margin for error is considerable. The responsibility on the doctor was enormous. There were probably hundreds of 'Violets' all over the country whose welfare and entire future, virtually life or death, was decided by the ward doctor. Those doctors were all young and, no matter how intelligent, their experience was in front of them and not behind them.

I began to observe the ward more closely and noticed how badly off everybody was for bed linen. Everything was patched and sheets coming back from the laundry could hardly hold together. The linen was also rough and coarse. The ward boasted of three Fowler beds. These were a new innovation used mainly after abdominal operations and very comfortable. But it was no use trying to settle down in those beds, for as soon as patients were slightly better they were shifted into ordinary beds which were hard, lumpy and uncomfortable. The most troublesome feature of the beds were thick, waterproof drawsheets, underneath the top sheet. Impossible to keep flat, these were always rucking up and caused great discomfort. Everyone had one of those thick, dark red, rubber drawsheets – Sister said these were imperative, as they saved the mattresses. Privately I thought of all the things it was possible to say about these mattresses, though that they might be saved was not included in the list. Bedsores were always a nightmare to staff and patients: in all fairness this could not always be avoided, however good the nursing. This ward had its quota of patients with bedsores, and in view of the lumpy mattresses, the rubber drawsheets and the inflated air-cushions with rigid edges, I wonder there were not more.

There was a passion in this ward for tucking patients in with the bedclothes, so that they could not move. Perhaps the aim of this exercise was for the beds to appear so flat and tidy as to give the impression there was no one inside them. After a round of such bedmaking, one could observe patients quietly wriggling in order to free their arms or, more difficult still, to fight for another few inches to make room for their toes. The methods used for freeing oneself varied. The younger and more agile patients used to do this in one fell swoop, with an upward heave of both elbows, together with both knees. Some of the more ill or older people used to secretly enlist the help of those up and about to release them. We felt we needed lessons in escapology. Twenty-six beds took quite some time to make even by the speediest nurses, so by the time the last of the beds had been made, a number of us had already managed to manœuvre ourselves into a position of greater freedom of movement. The nurses surveyed the ward after making all the beds and would usually emit shrieks of horror with the cry, 'Mrs – we have only just finished making the beds and look at you, all untidy again!'

This hospital was situated in a poor working-class area and had to contend with a lot of trouble due to drink. Bank holidays and their aftermath gave the doctors a great deal of extra work. There was always a certain amount of conversation amongst the staff as to what went on in Casualty during the night and Bank holidays were usually field nights. Nurse was making my bed one day following a Bank holiday, when the Casualty doctor came round to talk to her. She asked about Casualty during the night and he replied that it had been hectic. He told her a man had been brought in badly cut with a bottle during a brawl and he had to do a lot of stitching. Nurse then inquired as to whether he did this under anaesthetic, to which the doctor replied there had been absolutely no need, since the man was so drunk he did not feel anything. I could not help but listen to this conversation. The thought crossed my mind that perhaps getting drunk could be substituted for anaesthetics, as it somehow seemed a less violent way of becoming unconscious; I did not know at the time, this method was, in fact, used before the discovery of anaesthetics.

Conversations between members of the staff always continued as though the patients were not present. This same procedure was often employed when the patient was not only present but directly involved. Some doctors would deign to make some token remark to the patient, and others, particularly specialists in the voluntary hospitals, would not utter at all.

Nurses usually carried on a round of conversation whilst they made the beds and always talked shop. They talked in this fashion because hours were very long and, once on duty, they were rarely away from the ward. All nurses seemed to have more work than they could reasonably be expected to do, though the amount of work they did in this hospital wanted seeing to be believed. Nurses and Sister told me that they were sometimes too tired to go out when off-duty and, before going to sleep, would raise the foot of their beds and sleep like a log. I must stress such remarks were not made in a spirit of dissatisfaction or complaint but merely as a statement of fact. Nearly all the twenty-six people in this ward needed dressings and treatment. Directly after Sister's morning report the nurses began dressings and it was non-stop until lunchtime. Some dressings which were not sterile would be left until after lunch. Whilst the voluntary hospital nurses also worked very hard, there seemed to be more available. In those days the volume and pressure of work was enormous, as a large number of chores then included in the work for nurses are now done by ward orderlies. I used to wonder how many miles a day a nurse walked while on duty and if this had ever been computed.

Of the many outstanding nurses I recall on this ward, one in particular was quite amazing and made a life-long impression on me. She had come to this hospital a fully trained, State Registered staff nurse. Her system of work was so remarkable that present-day time and motion study experts might have learned a great deal. This nurse did all the dressings and treatment on this heavy ward, often on her own, with a rhythm of work that was a model of organized skill. Like all experts she never made an unnecessary movement or journey. Light of touch – and this can be a blessing to patients with raw and sore conditions – she was the personification of the Nightingale nurse, albeit without the status. Nurses trained in voluntary hospitals were considered on a higher level, possibly because the standard of entry was higher and there was a wider choice of student nurses. After several months on this ward, this particular nurse elected to go and work among the old people in the workhouse. The medical superintendent begged her to remain in the hospital. He actually came into the ward one day while she was working and said, 'Do you really want to go over the "other side"?' She replied, 'Yes, I like and feel sorry for old people and want to work among them.' I overheard this conversation myself. She was a very attractive young woman about twenty-six years old. So what the ward lost the destitute aged gained, and on weighing things up, their need was the greater.

Other nurses who made a lasting impression on me were those from the religious orders, who came to help out on night-duty. Without exception they were patient and kind. Quiet, by virtue of their religious training, their presence on the ward by night was both peaceful and efficient.

After I had been in this ward for a short time, something happened which might have ended very badly for me and, what is worse, something I could have prevented. It appeared that Milly had a bath twice a week in the big bath outside the ward. Nurse used to carry her to and from the bathroom, she was so light in weight. Milly much enjoyed those excursions and I was rather envious. Having similar complaints, Milly and myself were linked together in a curious way. The doctor and nurses often addressed us collectively beginning, 'Now then, you two.' There was the change-over of nurses on the ward and, as usual, the complaint and treatment of each patient was explained to the incoming nurses. I should hazard a guess for purposes of that explanation, Milly and myself were coupled together. The following day the new nurse gave Milly her bath as usual and later said to me, 'Now how much do you weigh – could I carry you? Being new on the ward she assumed I also would have a bath. I only had blanket baths and could not remember the last time I had been in a proper bath. Although I was well aware of this, the temptation to have an excursion to and from the bathroom was so great, I did not tell the nurse. New nurses on the ward often got details of procedure from the patients – it was really very naughty of me not to have said anything. Nurse carried me into the bathroom which I had never seen. It was a large, dreary-looking room. Comfortless, untidy and devoid of anything not strictly utilitarian. With a mottled stone floor, the walls painted dark green, the eternal red rubber sheets draped round the walls, two very old, wooden wheelchairs pushed into one corner it looked what it was – part of a charity institution. The bathroom looked as though it had been built on at a later date, since part of the roof contained a skylight which, together with the window, made it very light; so that it did have one saving grace. Not that any of those outward manifestations, good or bad, bothered me at all, for I never enjoyed a bath so much as I enjoyed that one.

It is difficult to explain to anyone who has not experienced it, what the feeling is like through being sick and sore from lying in bed – I mean lying in bed for really long periods. From time to time this feeling set up an irritation, a resentment and frustration for which, short of doing something desperate, there was no solution. The feeling passed though it sometimes lasted for days, until one came to terms again. I suppose this explanation could pass as a good and sufficient reason for the way in which I behaved, had not the consequences of this bath been so disastrous.

After the bath I arrived back in bed very pleased but also very breathless. I decided to relax and keep very quiet for a while, since the heat of the bath and all this unaccustomed movement proved a great exertion for me. The breathlessness became progressively worse until half an hour later I could only breathe with great difficulty. Milly became alarmed and called the nurse who, in turn, fetched the doctor. My temperature rose to 105° so the doctor suggested my having a tepid wash. True, I had been eager to have a bath though I did not bargain for two baths, as the tepid wash was really a second bath. With the help of oxygen, I was able to fight off this attack in the early hours of the morning. The doctor was naturally very nonplussed as to what caused this seizure and asked several leading questions. I feigned total ignorance though I was very worried in case the nurse got into trouble. Notwithstanding that the decision whether or no I should have a bath would never have been regarded as my responsibility, the fact remains that patients who have been in hospital a long time did become familiar with the routine and quite often gave useful information to the staff. It really was all my fault as a short explanation would have certainly made the nurse think again before giving me a proper bath.

The next day was Sunday. It was Sister's week-end off so that she was not around when the bath saga took place. This was to the good, as she had a habit of ferreting out certain facts and unearthing hidden stories. Sister was really a very stable person and not given to histrionic displays when things went wrong in the ward. However, she had two pet hates: one was cats and the other the Salvation Army.

Being a ground floor ward, cats would occasionally wander in, though they never got very far. Sister would appear as from nowhere and chase them out energetically, calling them nasty, dirty, germ-carrying pests. One day the ward patients were treated to an extraordinary diversion. Sister was alerted to the fact that a black cat had found its way into the ward. She immediately appeared carrying a broom with the avowed aim of chasing the cat out of the ward. The black cat took up the challenge and sprang with an agility that only cats possess, from one side of the ward to the other, winding her lithe, black body in and out of the bottom rails of the beds. Sister lunged at the animal to no avail. She was no match for the cat, who managed to avoid the broom and retain her position underneath one of the beds. Sister was seen to retire from the ward still carrying the broom. A few minutes later the cat emerged from under the bed, made a slow, dignified exit from the ward and was gone before Sister had time to return to the fray. Actually the black cat won the day.

Relations with the Salvation Army, however, were another matter.

Every Sunday morning without fail at 11 a.m., the Salvation Army gave a short religious service in the ward. There were usually two men and three women. They arrived complete with a small harmonium which was played by a rather large man, gave a short Bible reading, sang two hymns and were gone within ten minutes. So far as Sister was concerned this was ten minutes too long. If she happened to be on duty she would leave the ward the moment they arrived, muttering under her breath, and return as soon as they had departed. Personally, I did not mind the service and do not think anybody else objected. Why Sister disliked the Salvation Army remains an unfathomable mystery.

This was the only hospital where I saw the Salvation Army

take the Sunday service, though religion was always very much part of the scene, both in the council and voluntary hospitals. The amount of religion varied from the short, weekly service which I have just described to one voluntary hospital where I was a patient and prayers were held regularly, morning and evening; led by Sister or whoever was in charge, the nurses knelt down and prayed out loud, while many of the patients joined in. Voluntary hospitals have a powerful link with religion since their early history is bound up with the Church. The very word 'hospital' is a derivation of 'hospice'. All religious denominations were allowed into the ward and one day my attention was drawn to the fact that the Protestant, Catholic and Jewish ministers were all there at the same time. Many patients were visited by the minister of the Church they usually attended and mostly, though by no means in every case, a minister would come if a patient was dying.

On the routine round one morning after I had been in this hospital about five months, the doctor asked me whether I would chance another operation. He said that if what he had in mind was successful, it might give me a new lease of life; adding there was no particular hurry, he left it at that. Having mentioned the subject, the eternal dream of a quick recovery was now on my mind and I could think of little else. The doctor pursued the idea again the following week and explained the type of operation he suggested would have to be performed in two parts. He took a piece of writing paper from my bed-table and proceeded to make a sketch of what he intended to do. (Many years later, rummaging through old letters and papers, I found this very rough drawing, which would have conveyed nothing whatsoever to anyone else.) He stressed an operation of this kind was the only thing possible and he would explain the situation to Mother. From the stage of feeling hopeful, excited and elated, I now started to feel frightened and depressed. What if the operation was unsuccessful? I brushed aside this feeling. This reaction of depression was in no way connected with doubts about the doctor. As I have already said he was a big man who seemed to radiate confidence. I must confess I cannot think of any sound reason why size should be equated with skill and experience, but the fact remains that at no time did I doubt his ability to perform such an operation.

When Mother came to see me the following visiting day she was late and told me that the doctor had spoken to her about my having another operation. I sensed both Mother and myself shared the same thoughts, namely, I had no other alternative and I told the doctor so when he did the round next morning. It seemed I would have to wait for this operation, as the doctor wished to arrange it on a day when he could have the operating theatre to himself. The use of the theatre was planned among the various doctors and they performed their surgery on the same day each week. There must have been special arrangements for emergencies.

This particular doctor was very kind to me all the time he was at this hospital and was one of the very few doctors who did not treat me like a moron. Mostly, the attitude towards patients was, 'Take it or leave it', that there was no time to explain anything and, even if there was time, the patient would not understand anyway. I never accepted the reasons given for this approach. No. It was simply an attitude of mind towards certain classes of people. This did not apply to patients who went to see a doctor privately, for the doctor would ask if there were any questions he could answer. It is often said that the private patient receives no better treatment than the poorer one. This I would certainly concede. What is so different is the attitude; and this is what the doctor/patient relationship is all about. As a point of interest, there has been a great change in this kind of approach for people are now better educated and better informed, in spite of the glamorized versions of hospital life that sometimes appear on television. The 'hard line' is still maintained by some for tradition is slow to change, yet change there has been. I have heard the younger generation of doctors and nurses ridicule this attitude. It was neatly summed up by one of the nurses when I was recently in hospital who said (referring to one of the older specialists), 'He thinks he's God!'

I had this operation three weeks later on a day not used for general surgery and came out of it better than expected. To everyone's joy and most especially my own, the wound started to heal in – I could almost see it getting better. For the first time in years I was free of the everlasting pain. Everything proceeded as the doctor had foretold and five weeks later he suggested I might try to get out of bed. I almost over-reached myself in the effort to start walking, as I had not been up for a year and a half. I had the greatest difficulty in trying to remain calm and pretend everything was as usual. Trying to walk was not easy and I had quite a shock when, after various attempts, both my legs swelled up to about twice their normal size. Nevertheless, I did quite well and managed to keep my balance. This problem of maintaining balance was most awkward. Having been in bed so long I was not accustomed to look downwards, so that when I got up on my feet, I had the sensation of swaying, even when holding tight on to some immovable object. It was like being on board a ship, except that I could reasonably expect the ward not to move around.

Although I did not know this at the time, the doctor had applied for a post at another hospital. The first half, having been so successful, he quite understandably wished to complete this operation by doing the second half, so ten weeks later said I should have this other operation. I recall how strong was my desire to be left alone at that stage – at least for the time being. I told the doctor of my feelings on the matter and he thought I ran a grave risk by postponing the next operation. He spoke to me at great length and put me entirely at ease, by carefully explaining once again many of the things he had previously told me, insisting that the important part had already been done and what was about to happen was nothing by comparison. He never once hinted that the timing of this operation might have something to do with his leaving the hospital. With great restraint, I fought to overcome the feeling of digging my heels in and saying 'No'.

The doctor knew the frame of mind I was in since I made no secret of it and he then said something which he had not mentioned before. Having had a short circuit of the bowel I still had a mucus discharge, though this was no more than a nuisance. The doctor called my attention to the condition and added, 'If that suddenly became septic, peritonitis could set in immediately and I would not be able to save you.' My feelings were subjective and abstract, whilst the doctor had knowledge based on concrete, inside (literally) information. The lay person is in an impossible situation when it comes to problems of this nature so, much against my intuitive feelings, the operation was agreed. Having taken the decision I tried very hard to push aside all doubts and to look ahead. I argued with myself that, after all, my objection was based only on the timing of the operation. For reasons I was unable to explain, I simply felt I needed more time – this was the only ground upon which I wavered.

There were no special arrangements for this next operation which was performed on Wednesday, the routine surgery day. I remember very little of the week following, except that everything went wrong. The anaesthetic was a positive nightmare, as I kept vomiting and could not lose consciousness. This had never happened to me before; I was not surprised to learn later that I had a collapse under the anaesthetic. I am not qualified to comment as to why this happened, though I was worn down before the operation started. Perhaps by resisting the anaesthetic, I was trying to do what I really wanted, which was not to have had the operation at that particular time. Prior to the operation I certainly do not recall thinking in this way, for I was quite prepared to trust the doctor and accept his explanation. I went over all this in my own mind to try and find a solution, a rationale, as to why this operation, which was a secondary one, should have become so violent and ended so badly. I pulled through the first week and started to mend. Until then the surgery had seemed all right. It was my general condition which caused concern, so imagine the shock and consternation when, ten days after the operation had been performed, the wound completely gave way again and I found myself in a far worse situation than when I first arrived at this hospital.

For my own part, the feeling that I was now a hopeless case hit me like a thunderclap, since I had never before regarded myself as such. Something died in me that day and I lost a confidence which never returned. Even years after I was better, the uncertainty of what happened over those three weeks haunted me. At a time when people expected me to be on the very wings of happiness, I was glad not to talk or have to answer questions – after all, I had been almost better before.

Shortly after this the doctor left the hospital to go to his new post – I never saw him again. Nevertheless, I have always remembered him for a number of reasons. He took a genuine interest and wanted to make me better. He tried everything he knew to make this come about and was unable to hide his disappointment when things went so wrong. During the time I spent in hospital I must have seen scores of different doctors and he was the only one who asked whether my mother was able to bring me the things I needed in the way of extras. He mentioned this when I first came to the hospital and added, if I wished he could write me up for a number of things such as fruit or other goodies. I thanked him and replied that I managed to get by. This gesture, however, must be appraised in the light of existing circumstances.

All hospitals are very expensive to run. The ultimate objective of all those engaged on the organizational and social side, such as the chairman, secretaries and almoners, was to try and lessen the burden of expenditure. The voluntary hospitals ran a perpetual campaign to try and obtain more money and it was quite usual for wards to be temporarily shut down for lack of funds. The financial position of the newly constituted council hospitals was a kind of half-way measure. Their income was derived partly from local grants and partly from block grants from the exchequer. A percentage of money in all hospitals was collected from patients and this fell heavily on people of low income groups who happened to be ill. In voluntary hospitals the amount of payment was determined by the management, whilst the ability to pay was assessed by the almoner, a procedure which I have already described in the first chapter. The council hospitals also had special committees which sat for this purpose. There was, in fact, a means test for both groups of hospitals. With widespread unemployment it was impossible for large numbers of patients to pay at all. Local council hospitals supplied medical necessities and basic meals. Certain extras could be obtained if the doctor thought it necessary. Patients having to rely entirely on hospital food may not have starved though the meals were meagre and badly cooked, so that by no stretch of the imagination could the ordinary hospital diet be considered as part of the cure. Only since the Act of 1948 have patients been able to subsist completely on the diet supplied, without having to rely on food being brought in. Therefore, when the doctor kindly suggested he could get me some extras, it must be considered against the background of the times.

Milly and myself did have some unofficial concessions with regard to food. I noticed when I first arrived that Milly's family often brought in cooked meals for her. I inquired whether this was allowed, to which question Milly replied in her forthright fashion, 'Of course it's not allowed, but if your mother can manage it Sister will turn a blind eye.' I promptly took up this cue and asked my mother if she could bring me something home cooked. The very next visiting day she arrived with a small chicken dinner, complete with baked potatoes. This was no mean feat, since we lived a considerable distance from the hospital, so that the meal had to be heavily insulated to keep it warm. Mother made me laugh when she told me how she sat quietly in the bus with the hot dinner in a basket on her lap. After a while the succulent odour of roast started to circulate round the bus and how one of the passengers said, 'What a lovely smell, it makes me feel hungry.' I told Mother this was an unsolicited testimonial to her good cooking.

Following this last deplorable operation I entered a new phase. The attitude of the new ward doctor was one of resignation – that is, like Milly, here I was and here I was likely to remain. My own attitude was bad, inasmuch as I lost a great deal of my usual fight and seemed to be losing the battle against slow decline and the feeling of wilting. Some mornings when the doctor came to do the round I pretended to be asleep – we had nothing to say to each other. In reply to the routine question of, 'How are you today?' I could either answer that I was better which was not so, or else I could say I was just the same, which did not mean anything. Mostly I chose to say nothing and feigned sleep. Not so Milly, who always had lengthy conversations with the doctor about the weather, the news, about almost anything except the reason for her being in hospital. Not that she did not want to get better. It was simply that she refused to indulge in wishful thinking, and in this way appeared to have come to terms with the existing circumstances. Although my attitude seemed one of despair at the time, it contained also the bitter regret, the dissatisfaction and unrest, which made it impossible for me to come to terms. Therein lay the difference between Milly and myself, in spite of the temporary loss of mood following the unsuccessful operation.

One day, in a fit of depression, I complained to Milly and asked, 'Why do you think the doctor does not bother about us at all? Is it that he does not know of any treatment he might try, or that we are just written off as a loss and no one will ever bother about us again?' Milly replied very briskly, 'You realize he could make us worse by trying out the wrong things – or even kill us off. After all,' she continued, 'I've had no end of surgery and treatment and you are not far behind and where has it got us? Nowhere.'

I found it difficult to come to terms with Milly's argument, though I had to admit it was based on commonsense. Milly went on as though trying to convince herself, 'It's really best to try not to think or talk about it.' Milly then added, as though divining my thoughts, 'Although in reality I know it's impossible to pretend the problem does not exist.' I pressed forward with my own ideas and said to Milly, 'Are there many days or more especially nights, when you don't pause to consider this eternal problem?' Milly then made a rare admission by saying, 'Well, I do think about it most days but don't talk about it.' This was probably the truth of the matter for she never of her own free will started a conversation of this kind and it was one of the very rare moments when she let herself go in this way. Milly was very quick tempered and by no means a phlegmatic type, so that she must have thought the matter out and decided discussions of this nature could not lead anywhere – there was no point in thinking out loud.

Curiously enough a couple of days later, during the morning round, the doctor said to me, 'I would like you to try something out which may be uncomfortable, but no more.' I wondered what was coming. The doctor continued, 'I would like you to have solids only for a few days and not to drink at all, except for an occasional sip of cold water.' This was something quite new – I had never before heard of such treatment, though I readily agreed to faithfully co-operate as from the next day. In theory it sounded relatively simple – in practice it was awful. I started off by forgoing the early morning tea and likewise having no tea with my breakfast. Sister also seemed a trifle mystified by this line of treatment and instructed the nurse to leave me plenty of mouthwash, so as to counter the feeling of dryness. By the end of the first day I could have cheerfully drunk all the mouthwash disinfectant. Milly said, 'The doctor must have overheard our conversation and thought out something to do.' By the end of the second day, I told Sister I did not think that I could continue much longer and asked whether she knew what result was supposed to be achieved by this treatment. Sister was very guarded in her reply, 'I'm sure the doctor knows what he's about.' I was never so pleased to see the ward doctor as I was at the end of that third day, when I told him I felt I must have a drink of some kind. The doctor readily agreed. 'Oh yes, return to normal diet.' Milly was distinctly amused at this episode. 'Of course, I can afford to laugh, but it is funny coming so soon after our conversation about feeling neglected.' I told Milly we might set about compiling a dictionary of strange treatments and that this could be placed alongside the egg-white treatment when I first arrived. I must add I also came over a little further to Milly's viewpoint, that it was sometimes better to be ignored.

The head doctor in this hospital was known as the medical superintendent. Milly and myself knew him by sight. He walked through the ward occasionally though he never had any direct contact with the patients. He was a dark man of medium height, with a short clipped moustache and a pair of shrewd, penetrating eyes that never seemed to miss anything. He was always very correctly dressed and looked like a top grade civil servant, without the briefcase or umbrella.

One afternoon he walked through the ward with Sister and stopped between Milly's bed and my own. Milly, as usual, was crocheting for her pincushions and I was staring into space. He looked at Milly and myself very intently for a few seconds and then uttered one sentence. He said, 'Sister, those two girls ought to be in the "House" – they just occupy two beds to no purpose.' Like Madame Defarge knitting in *A Tale of Two Cities*, Milly went on with her crochet and I continued to stare into space. But we both heard very clearly what the medical superintendent had said.

Having spoken the awful sentence, the superintendent walked out of the ward with Sister. I had never seen Milly so agitated. She hastily put away her work and asked me whether I had understood him correctly. I replied that I quite understood him, but what did the 'House' mean? Milly gave me a withering look and almost shouted 'The workhouse, of course' – I gathered the impression that she added 'you fool'. It was my turn to look startled. I asked incredulously, 'Could he really do such a thing as take us out of the ward and put us in the workhouse?' Milly assured me that he was empowered to do this and proceeded to pose a number of rhetorical questions. How could we prevent ourselves from being seized and taken out of the ward? What steps were possible should the porter suddenly arrive and try and take us without warning? Should we tell our families or tackle the situation ourselves? etc. I simply had to have time to think about all this – I was completely staggered and had no idea such a move was possible. It was alarming. I started to try and sort the matter out logically. I mentally argued after all, if the voluntary hospitals were able to get rid of their long-stay and chronic sick patients by putting them into the recently constituted council hospitals the logical conclusion seemed to be, there was nothing to stop the council hospitals from passing their patients on to the workhouse.

Neither Milly nor I slept much that night and the night-nurse asked what was the matter with the pair of us. We did not go into explanations with her, because we were rather mixed up ourselves. Neither of us had ever been inside the workhouse: we had only seen two women who came from there and used to come into the ward occasionally. They were both dressed in the most peculiar grey, shapeless garments, which must have been the workhouse uniform. They seemed old, though they might not have been, since the clothes they were obliged to wear could have reduced the most fashion-conscious beauty to a freak. One of the patients was apparently known to them and they used to sit and chat with her. I had no idea of what the inmates were really like and tended to gaze on them like people from another planet. It might have been interesting to have known more about some of them. For example, I once heard the doctor tell Sister that he intended to go across to the 'House', to practise his French with somebody there. My curiosity was aroused when I heard the doctor say that, and later asked Sister who it was he went to see. Sister was not quite certain but thought it was an old lady who had once been a governess and was bi-lingual in French. The dread of being in the workhouse had been handed down from generation to generation for the last hundred years, so that whilst our actual experience of the workhouse was nil, we dreaded the thought because of its historical associations and dreaded still more the stigma by implication of having descended to the lowest of all social categories. However, what the medical superintendent had once again clearly brought out in that one sentence, was the utter hopelessness of our situation.

'Nice of the superintendent to plan for our future,' were Milly's first words next morning and then added, 'I have also been making plans.' She then elaborated by saying that whatever happened we should not go quietly but make as much fuss as possible and not to mind the other patients, as they would go home and we could not. She further suggested if we were pushed out and put into the workhouse by force, we were to make ourselves a continual nuisance by categorically refusing to co-operate with anything or anybody. I was rather uncertain as to how all this would work out in practice and thought we might need some other kind of help. I considered the possibility of appealing to Sister or the ward doctor. Milly was of the opinion that the power of the medical superintendent was such it could override everyone else, and other people could do nothing once we were in there. It was up to us. In the meantime we agreed to try not to go to sleep at the same time, as we thought it safer for one of us to be alerted. We both became more ill than we already were with worrying, though we said nothing to our families.

All this took place shortly before Christmas. As the days passed and nothing happened, Milly and myself simmered down a little and thought perhaps the powers high up had decided to leave the matter over until after Christmas, though we both continued to feel worried and unsettled.

Something occurred in the hospital during Christmas and the

New Year which seemed entirely unconnected with the question of our being moved into the workhouse. It was something which must have given the medical superintendent a great deal of worry and trouble. Milly said she was certain this incident so threw the superintendent off-guard, that he forgot or gave up the idea of moving us.

What happened was this.

Before Christmas it was usual for as many patients to go home as possible, and all ward sisters planned along those lines. Though some went home, the majority of nurses and doctors remained in the hospital to do what they could to make the Christmas holiday more cheerful. On Christmas Eve a group of nurses, headed by Matron and carrying lighted lanterns, sang carols. The ward was decorated with coloured balloons, paper chains, bells, silver tinsel and, on one side, was a paper rainbow ending in a pot of gold. This theme was devised and organized by Sister. The doctors put on a show for Christmas Day, which included a staff nurse and doctor who had changed clothes and did the ward round impersonating each other: this was very well done and proved hilarious. Christmas dinner had been a great success, so had the high tea which followed in the afternoon. In the early evening the Staff congregated in the side-ward, which was empty because the patient had been able to go home. (The side-ward was a large room with one bed, used for people with suspected infectious diseases, or those seriously ill.) The sounds of laughter and merrymaking could be heard not only from our floor, but from the floor above. However, everything could be well organized and planned in advance – except death.

As I have already explained, I was in a ground floor ward and the two wards above were for men. Needless to say I had never been upstairs and might have known nothing whatever about the men's wards had it not been for the Christmas celebrations. These jollifications used to carry on beyond the New Year because the staff was very large and not everybody could celebrate at the same time The side-wards must have been empty, as we could all hear sounds of a gramophone playing upstairs and a muffled sound of shuffling feet, as though people were dancing. Snatches of a popular song could be heard called 'Dancing with

Tears in my Eyes': this record seemed to be played on the gramophone over and over again

Just after Christmas, whispered comments percolated through to the ground floor ward. Milly and I both sensed there was something wrong in the hospital, though we did not know what it was. Nothing out of the ordinary had occurred in the ward which we were in though it seemed certain that something had happened on this block. Milly made discreet inquiries but could find out nothing. She was always interested in hospital scandal, claiming that it created a diversion and made life more interesting. No doubt, a great deal did go on in the hospital, though very little information came the way of the patients. Although Milly was on the scent, there were no definite clues. I suggested perhaps the rumours were untrue and that nothing had happened. Milly's reply was characteristic for she said, 'I feel sure something so awful has happened that nobody dare discuss it openly!'

Milly was right. Something awful had happened.

Two weeks later I received the one and only anonymous communication I have ever received in my life. It contained a letter and a copy of a weekly newspaper named *John Bull*. The paper was folded in such a way as to show an article headed in large bold type which read, 'HOSPITAL DEATH DANCE'. On the top left-hand corner of this page was a gloomy picture of the black, iron gates, at the main entrance of the hospital. In this picture the gates looked even more prison-like than the reality. I am able to recall the content of this article in some detail – it was shattering.

In the men's ward upstairs a man on the danger list was visited by his wife and sister at five-thirty one afternoon. In the next bed, which was screened off, another patient named Mr Brooks lay dying. A few yards away from the ward a dance was in progress; the article stressed that the gramophone seemed to be continuously playing a song called, 'I'm Dancing with Tears in my Eyes', the tune which we in the ground floor ward also heard. The dancers consisted of nurses and male attendants, who sometimes danced from the corridor into the ward. A nurse, sitting with the dying patient, Mr Brooks, emerged three times from behind the screen to inquire from the visitors whether the time was yet 6 p.m.

At 6 p.m. prompt, the nurse left the ward. The dying man was quiet. Ten minutes later the man gave an agonizing scream and wailed for nearly ten minutes. Nobody came near him. The wife and sister visiting the man in the next bed could no longer bear the screams and went out of the ward in search of a nurse. The dancing was still in progress and they stopped one of the nurses in the middle of a two-step to tell her about the man who was screaming. The nurse listened, checked with the two women as to who the patient was and then said, 'Nonsense, that man is dead – he died at 6 p.m.' The visitors protested the man was calling for help and the nurse insisted that he was dead. The two visitors returned to the ward, went behind the screen and saw the man with his eyes open and breathing. For a short time all was quiet. The man then started to wail again and sounded as though he was vomiting. The noise of a basin clattering towards the floor was heard – it seemed the dying man had tried to reach a basin and failed. The two visitors once again went into the corridor and asked another nurse to have a look at the man The nurse protested at being asked though she did go into the ward and stayed a matter of seconds with the dying Mr Brooks, after which she too left the ward. A few minutes later the dying man groaned and gasped. One of the ward patients went behind the screen and came out saying, 'Brooks is dead.' The time was 6.30 p.m. The visitors again went in among the dancers and told them the patient had died. On hearing this, a party of them rushed into the ward and went behind the screen. The man was dead – he had died at 6.30 p.m. and not at 6 o'clock as reported.

When the nurses came out from behind the screen, one of them said to the visitors and other patients who witnessed the scene, 'Mind your own business.'

The next morning one of the visitors returned to the ward. She was the wife of the man on the danger list, and demanded that her husband be taken home. The doctor told her this was a very grave step, since he had only one chance in a hundred of living. His wife insisted she wanted him to have that chance at home, not in a hospital where she had seen such awful things. The man was taken home.

When he arrived home, he asked that a reporter be sent for

from this weekly newspaper. The reporter came to the house and the man told him all he, his wife and sister-in-law had seen at the hospital. The reporter checked on the facts which were found to be true and wrote them up as an article for his paper. It was in effect a deathbed statement for, some days later, this man who was in the next bed to the unfortunate Mr Brooks, also died.

The weekly paper, *John Bull*, which reported these facts was very well known and enjoyed a large, national circulation. It has only recently ceased publication. Milly and I never heard how far the repercussions of this article went except, according to the paper, that a member of the London County Council called for 'vigorous, official action'.

So much for the content of the article.

The anonymous letter enclosed with the weekly also made a startling revelation. The letter started by stating I might be interested to read the article and also to learn that it was impossible to buy this paper for miles around. It was known that a doctor from this hospital had bought up every available copy. The letter ended with kind regards to Milly and myself, wishing us both well and, of course, minus a signature. We never discovered who sent it. The only identification was the handwriting, which was good, and the local postmark.

Milly quite rightly observed that buying up all the available copies of the paper containing this article must have cost a great deal of time and money. She was firmly convinced that organizing such a widespread campaign must have put everything else out of the mind of the medical superintendent, including the plan to move Milly and myself into the workhouse. It is uncertain whether these two incidents concerning the medical superintendent were linked, though it certainly created an interesting chain of events. Milly and myself remained in the same ward and heard no more about going into the workhouse.

During the winter months, pressure on the hospital became so great that extra beds were placed down the middle of the ward. Sometimes the children's ward became full and it was during one such crowded period that a little girl was put into this ward. She was made much of by the other patients and also the doctor, who was fond of children. Her name was Joan and she was seven years old. Most children were very unhappy at being separated from their mother. This did apply to Joan at the beginning of her five weeks' stay in the ward, but she soon settled down and gave us all the benefit of her very quaint opinions. Two incidents were really amusing. She appeared very preoccupied one afternoon and finally called the staff nurse to inquire, 'If the sister was a sister was the doctor a brother?' The other story was connected with the hospital heating system, which was always inadequate in cold weather. The ward was never warm enough. This was due to the open passage ways which I described earlier. The ward doors were insufficient protection against the gusts of wind which circulated through those open corridors. The ward radiators were forever being adjusted in the hope they would throw out more heat. Following one such adjustment the radiator started leaking. A large pool of water soon collected on the floor. The doctor, walking round with Joan on his usual morning round, noticed the water and, commenting on the obvious, said, 'The radiator must be leaking.' To this Joan promptly agreed adding, 'No one could have done all that!'

When Joan was discharged her mother had some difficulty in persuading her to come home. She said she liked it in hospital and wanted to stay. After some further discourse on the matter between Joan, her mother and Sister she announced she would, after all, go home, and left the ward amid goodbyes, kisses and bearing masses of toys.

The new ward doctor was a Scot, with a very deep brogue and a shy manner. The first time he saw me he asked detailed questions about the pain, which was there virtually all the time. He said he would put me on a drug which I could have at night or any time I felt unable to cope. To me this was an entirely new approach. I had taken the usual quota of morphine and other drugs which were given after major operations and never remember thinking about them afterwards or being able to distinguish any specific after-effects. The drug prescribed by the doctor was called Nepenthe, which I think is one of the opium group. It was a thick liquid, dark brown in colour and tasted very bitter. The amount I drank was only a few drops at the bottom of a medicine glass, yet, for the first time I experienced what the after-effects of drugs could really be like. I experienced for the first time, the feeling of coming out of myself as it were and floating in mid-air. The distinct feeling of my being two selves, one static and the other floating, created a feeling of enchantment and ecstasy. It was difficult to gauge how long this amazing feeling lasted – it might only have been a matter of seconds. But it has made me better understand what it is that makes the modern craze for drugs so fascinating and desired by certain people, that they will go almost to any length to obtain them. What I find less easy to comprehend is what makes a drug habit forming. There were two very distinct stages. I was on Nepenthe for two years and what to my mind overshadows the rapture of the first stage, were the quite appalling after-effects of the second. Following the first pleasurable feeling, I would have a few hours very heavy sleep and awake with the awful feeling of being weighted down with lead, literally unable to raise my head off the pillow. It was a struggle to enter the conscious world. For want of a better description I used to call this a headache, though it was really much worse than the most severe headache I ever experienced. This lasted the whole of the next day, so that when I took this drug it actually took me some thirty hours to recover from one dose. Although pain was entirely shut out during this period, I did not take this drug if I could possibly carry on without it. If the first reaction was ecstatic, the far longer effects of leaden dullness and stupor were destroying. It was the choice of two evils.

In later years I thought about that period and wondered why I never became used to the drug and addicted – the opportunity seemed to be there. True, I did take it when it was available to me, though, even as I drank it, I was always first haunted by the vision of the dismal after-effects. I came off this drug very suddenly when I left the hospital and do not recall being unduly troubled. Perhaps there is a difference between those who take drugs for physical and emotional sensation and those who take them as a respite from pain?

There were all manner of difficulties for patients in hospital. No less, however, for the families of the chronic sick, though these were of a different kind. There was the question of expense; with fares to pay, food to buy, personal laundry to attend to and most visitors brought flowers, this was a consideration. Moreover, there was the overwhelming sense of obligation, with the thought in mind of how dreadful it seemed for one to be in hospital and have nobody to come and see them. I well remember Mother coming to see me in all weathers and when she was really ill herself, as she could not bear the thought of my not having a visitor. Short-term patients usually had their friends and families to see them – there was no problem. It was the chronic sick who found the circle of visitors become fewer, until only the immediate family came regularly. In the case of young people such as Milly and myself, we started in hospital as teenagers and grew away from our friends, because they had developed under normal conditions.

It was a kind of unwritten law that Milly and myself never discussed the future. We lived from day to day. Sometimes an echo from the world outside would project itself and set us thinking. This happened when an old friend came to see me unexpectedly. I remembered her at school as carefree, somewhat scatterbrained, with a fixed idea of becoming a famous ballroom dancer. During those three years I had not seen her, she was so changed I could not conceal my astonishment. It was not so much physical as other changes, for she had become calm, assured and very grown-up. I asked her whether she had taken up ballroom dancing and she went off into peals of laughter. 'My dear,' she said, 'I am marrying a man who can't dance a step, and am busy flat hunting.' It seemed I was the only one who remembered her crush on ballroom dancing. When she left I said to Milly, 'That girl had a strange effect on me, I don't know why.' 'I know why,' explained Milly by way of reply, 'it's because she talked about the world with a future – not the kind of world that we live in.'

Many patients could have gone out during the day or home for short periods. I once asked Sister why those able to go out were not allowed to do so. Sister maintained that the hospital authorities were responsible for all patients under their care and there were difficulties once patients were outside the hospital precincts. This was nonsense. Many people in hospital now go home for the week-end or out during the day and there is nothing to prove this dangerous or detrimental. In fact, it is to the good, since it mitigates against the claustrophobic feeling of being 'institutionalized'. Again, it was the attitude of the time. People in hospital were not merely the sick being treated, but the hospital authorities possessed them body and soul. Of course, it was possible for patients to discharge themselves. I had often seen this happen and did so myself, though patients unable to do this were, in fact, prisoners. Milly and myself could have been taken out for short periods by some method of conveyance. Had some kind person volunteered to do this, it would have been disallowed. Happily, this approach has also changed.

Occasionally something occurred in the world outside the hospital to take us out of ourselves and the ward conversation entered a rare phase – that of current affairs. Such an incident took place on an October day in 1930, when the ill-fated airship *R101* passed over the hospital. At the time there was considerable controversy with regard to this airship, for some experts contended it was not airworthy. The *R101* was on its way to India. It crossed London, bound for the English Channel, where it ran into very bad weather and finally exploded trying to land in France. There were no survivors. Following this tragedy which shook the nation, no more aircraft of that type was built in Britain. At the time the airship passed over the hospital it created tremendous excitement in the ward. All those able went to the windows to watch the giant airship pass and as my bed was directly in front of a window, I had a particularly good view. As the *R101* receded from sight, I leaned further and further out of bed to catch a last glimpse with the result that when the massive airship finally disappeared, I over-balanced and was in danger of falling out of bed; I had to ask for help and was hauled back by some of the other patients.

About the same time there was a very sad event at the hospital. During the night one of the nurses had died of pneumonia and the ward doctor had been up all night in a vain effort to save her life. I might have known nothing of this, had not the two nurses making my bed mentioned it. They mentioned her by name – Nurse Carberry – and I remembered her on night duty. That a service was held for her during the following week and was attended by all the staff able to go, was a piece of information Milly had obtained from Sister. I was surprised that Sister went so far as to tell Milly anything like that, for there was always a great wall of secrecy surrounding anything which happened to the staff. Milly was, of course, an expert at obtaining information. She had an interesting knack of putting the right questions to the right people, sometimes with great success. By way of example, there was the unusual tale of the good-looking hospital porter.

One of the hospital porters was young and extremely handsome; a fact which, in its way, proved to be a great disadvantage, for it was not that he had a roving eye for the ladies as that women, young and not so young, could not help giving him a second look. He was actually the theatre porter and I never discovered his real name as he was known to staff and patients as Fairy. He was married to a respectable, young, working-class woman whose major preoccupation seems to have been watching that her husband did not stray from the straight and narrow path. Fairy, in the course of his duty, came into the ground floor ward quite often and he never failed to give Milly a wave or acknowledgement of some description. While waiting for one of the patients in the ward one day, he managed to have a quick, confidential chat with Milly and I could not help but notice how worried he looked. I afterwards said to Milly, 'What's the matter with Fairy, he does not look particularly happy?' Milly said, 'Between ourselves, he told me he was having wife trouble.' He said that his wife was in a continuous state of mounting suspicion and had apparently arrived at the point where she considered her husband as shiftless, faithless and thoroughly untrustworthy. Moreover, she considered her husband as one whose life was made up of perpetual, secret love affairs with women unknown. Milly was very attractive and had been engaged to be married before she became ill, so that I regarded her as the last word in sophistication on matters of matrimony. Milly considered the position of Fairy very serious, and told me his good looks would be his undoing. Being very naïve in such matters I said, 'Do you really think he has affairs with women?' To which Milly replied, 'It really doesn't matter whether it's true or not, because being as good-looking as he undoubtedly is, his wife will have to get used to the idea that girls can't leave him alone, or else they won't be able to stay together.' A short time after this Milly again confided in me. It seemed that the wife of Fairy had been up to the hospital and made a terrific scene and openly accused her husband of being false. At this point Milly lowered her voice and whispered, 'His wife actually slapped him in public.' Having been brought up in a family where jobs and earning capacity were always uncertain, I said to Milly, 'Do you think this will affect his job here?' Milly said she did not know and had not thought about that side of the problem. As a matter of fact, Fairy stopped coming into the ward and thereafter we did not see him. Milly tried very hard to find out all that had really happened, though never succeeded in getting the entire story. One day she said to the staff nurse, 'Staff, do you know what's become of Fairy, we never see him now?' Staff nurse then paid him the highest compliment of the times when she said, 'He's probably gone to Hollywood to become a film star.'

Another time Milly got to know that the ward doctor had been found in the corridor in a collapsed condition one morning. On receiving this news I sounded a trifle doubtful as I said, 'Do you think it's true?' Milly looked at me somewhat peeved as she considered I was casting aspersions on her sources of information. 'Of course it's true – all the doctors are thoroughly overworked and can only carry on the long hours of duty by taking stuff to help keep them awake.' Milly continued, 'I reckon the ward doctor took too much of something and it had the opposite effect on him.'

I observed during the time I was in hospital, and have noticed since, that the medical and allied professions have a rather strange attitude towards illness when it comes to themselves. I read a passage recently in which a doctor wrote, 'There is no one more pathetic than a sick doctor.' The interesting part of the sentence was the use of the word 'pathetic', which was not intended as an expression of sympathy, but almost as a condemnation or censure. It made me recall an incident one day while I was in this hospital. It was an evening when the ward was short staffed. Both Sister and the second-year nurse were off duty at the same time, which left the staff and junior nurses to look after the ward. This meant that all the evening treatment and dressings had to be done by the staff nurse. As she went round the ward to the various patients disappearing and reappearing in and out of the screens, I noticed how flushed she looked. When she came to me I asked her whether she felt all right; she confided in me that she felt awful and could hardly keep going. It seemed unwise to try and carry on since she was obviously ill, so I asked why she did not report sick. I remember her exact reply. She said, 'You don't understand – it's a disgrace for a nurse to be ill, so as soon as I'm off duty I'll take something and I'll be all right in the morning.' Her answer puzzled me though I did not say any more. Next morning I knew something was wrong because a new staff nurse was sent on to the ward. Information concerning the staff was difficult to come by, but I had many friends among the nurses and so found out that the previous staff nurse had contracted scarlet fever and had been taken to an isolation hospital on the very night I spoke to her. She was away for a long time. Quarantine was a state in which all the patients lost out since no visitors at all were allowed inside the ward for two weeks and we all felt like prisoners who had lost their remission – not to speak of the frustration of those about to be discharged who were unable to go home. This had already happened twice before due to patients having caught fevers though luckily this time there were no repercussions.

It was very much the exception for me to be able to give Milly some news as it was nearly always the other way about, so that when I told her she posed a purely academic question in the following way. 'Now I'm jolly glad we're not in quarantine, but I wonder what's the difference between a fever contracted by a staff nurse, as opposed to a fever contracted by a patient?'

Nurses might wear the same uniform, though underneath they were very different people. As the hospital was for many years my home, I tended to be free-and-easy in my relationship with the nurses, sometimes forgetting that the hospital was an impersonal institution that could never be a substitute for home. All the ward patients had temperatures taken morning and evening, but some were on four-hourly charts. The amount of time allowed for the thermometer to give the required result varied between a matter of seconds, to an unspecified time because the nurse taking temperatures had departed to do another job, thus forgetting the patient and the thermometer. I was having a chat with one of the second-year nurses whose name was Baker: she was taking the four-hourly temperatures and waiting for the thermometer to 'cook', as she called it. The conversation was discursive and finally worked round to hopeless conditions. There was nothing morbid about the conversation, so that when Nurse said to me, 'What would you do if you became convinced that an illness was hopeless?' I replied rather lightheartedly, 'Good heavens, never to be able to get out and about on my own steam – let me see, I might do myself in.'

Several weeks after that conversation, following the doctor's round, my notes were left on my bed. I never bothered about my notes, since by that time there was little I did not know about myself, apart from the medical terminology. Needless to say, I had completely forgotten about the conversation with Nurse Baker. But my attention was caught by a few words written on my notes and underlined with red ink which read, 'This patient has threatened to do herself in.' I was absolutely horrified. Firstly, nothing was further from my mind when I made this reply to Nurse Baker's question. Secondly, the law at that time made attempted suicide a punishable offence. All this arose from an inconsequential, rather flippant conversation. I could not say anything since medical notes were not supposed to be read by the patient. There and then I took the decision to destroy the offending page in my notes. I regarded the whole episode as an untrue twist to words never intended as a serious statement. It was an unguarded reply given to a deliberately phrased question. The problem was how to destroy this page? Although I always felt lonely, I was never alone. I had to wait months, though eventually an opportunity presented itself.

The opportunity came during a blanket-bath session. Nurse got everything ready; my bed was screened off, my pillows were put on one side, she brought the usual enamel bowl containing about three inches of warm water, under-blanket, soap, sponge and towel, etc., when Sister sent word she wished to see her. Nurse rolled down her sleeves, replaced her white, stiff cuffs and departed to see Sister. Left alone, I had no idea of how long she would be gone. After a few minutes I managed to ask Milly, through the screens, whether she could see Nurse. There was no sign of her and Milly said she would let me know when she saw her coming. I thought swiftly, if I want to get hold of my notes, it is now or never. Unfortunately, my notes hung on a wall hook above my bed and just out of reach. I retrieved my pillows on which I worked my way upwards to the top of the bed and with the aid of a writing pad, managed to get the notes down off the wall. I hastily picked out the page I wanted and hid it beneath the blanket. However, I was unable to get the notes back again on to the wall and in my fruitless efforts to accomplish this, I dropped them on to the floor. I said to Milly, 'Is there anybody up, I need some help.' Milly called to a young woman walking around in the ward, she came behind the screen and obligingly picked the notes up off the floor and replaced them on the wall hook. I had just enough time to stuff the page into the back of my locker when Nurse reappeared and said, 'Dear, dear, the water's quite cold, I'll have to get some more.'

When I took this page from the rest of my notes, it also included all kinds of other information since the pages were used on both sides. It was never missed.

The above incident reminded me of a teacher I once had, who was a very mild-mannered man. On the question of notes, however, he became rabid. Although he grudgingly admitted some notes were useful, he also stoutly maintained that reams of unnecessary notes were written, taking untold time to compile, which nobody ever read and were mostly a waste of effort. This was long before the computer age in which, in all probability, he would not have survived. There appeared to be a modicum of truth in his attitude with regard to my medical notes. These were a collection of years of data which nobody ever read. Theoretically, when the nurses had time they were supposed to study the patients' notes in order to learn more about them. The short answer to this was, the nurses never had time. The only thing the staff ever looked at were the top couple of pages and if there was vital information underneath, nobody ever bothered. In order to study my notes – or Milly's, which were even longer – it would have taken weeks to digest. It seemed that no one ever thought of wasting time in that way. No doubt my old teacher would have felt vindicated. This incident had another salutary effect on me; it made me very cautious as to what I said to people in a position to take it down in notes.

Time dragged by, and the months I was in bed now added up to years. When I first arrived at this hospital, it came as a shock when Milly told me she had been in bed over four years; but the time lag between us seemed to be narrowing. Things appeared to be at a standstill and if we did not get worse, we certainly did not get better. Many people who knew Milly, myself included, commented on the fact that she did not behave like an invalid, but maintained an interest in what was happening generally and in her personal appearance, right to the end. If Milly did not behave like an invalid, neither did I look like one. On the rare occasions I was visited by another doctor (usually an acquaintance of the ward doctor) there was invariably the same comment, namely, that it was difficult to believe, looking at me, that I had been ill for such a long time.

Later on, this difference between the way I looked and the grim reality of things as they were, stood me in good stead.

Even in adversity it is possible to count one's blessings. My greatest blessing was certainly the endless thought which my family – most especially my mother – gave to me in an effort to find a way which might make me better and so get me out of bed and hospital. When one is a teenager mums are very much taken for granted and I was no exception. But as I became older, and on looking back, it was little short of a miracle of devotion which my mother performed with no money and certainly no influence.

One visiting time Mother told me she had been discussing my situation at home and had come to the conclusion that unless something else was attempted, there seemed to be little chance of my getting better. As this hospital had obviously written me off this 'something' to which Mother referred would clearly have to come from outside. The problem was how to set about this? Whom to go to? This wound was now in a pretty hopeless state with a bowel perforated and blood, pus and fecal matter pouring through my side. Of course, I had seen a specialist before when I was able to go home, but my condition was now much worse. I was unable to walk and could not possibly go home.

This was the second time Mother was to obtain a medical opinion for me and she did this although on the first occasion the result had been calamitous, for no surgeon, however great, is infallible. Now she was doing this again, and not only what she did was of interest but also how she did it.

Mother first conferred with the family as to possible ideas and several lines of inquiry were started from home. Suggestions were made, some of which were totally impracticable, and others which came to nothing. For example, we had a very kindly, elderly family doctor who had known us for years and one of the suggestions was for Mother to discuss my position with him. This Mother did and said that he was very sympathetic though not co-operative.

Apparently he did not think it a good idea to start anything moving on the grounds it was extremely doubtful as to whether another consultant would wish to attempt anything further, and also the seriousness of likely repercussions in the event of failure. In short, he thought it was too risky, lest worse befall me.

Mother entered one of her profound thinking sessions, during which time she literally thought about a given situation by day and by night. She told me what the doctor at home had said and asked me point blank whether I wanted to give up the idea and said that, if not, she would have another go, since she had thought of another idea. For my own part I would have agreed to anything with the ghost of a chance of success, so that I felt pleased that Mother still wanted to keep trying. Mother next asked me to write out what I knew about myself and send it on to her, as she wished to show this to another doctor she intended to go and see. I then spent an enormous amount of time and effort as to how much I could leave out of this prepared statement without creating a false impression. I conferred with Milly who agreed it would be fatal to tell an outside doctor the stark and unadorned truth and urged me to stress the fact that I looked well in myself and to make the report sound generally gay and cheerful. Apparently the information served its purpose and I must confess I was rather flattered, when Mother later told me the doctor asked whether I had been a nurse at any time.

Mother put her idea into practice in the following way.

In the east end of London there was an organization called 'The Christian Medical Mission to the Jews', the basic objective of which was to convert Jews to Christianity. In charge of this mission was a Doctor Rocha (I think this was his name but I was never sure if Mother got it right) renowned as a good and conscientious doctor. Although I cannot recall any converts being made, there was no doubt that Doctor Rocha was much respected by a large number of Jewish people, and it was from him that Mother sought advice on whom to see and what to do about myself. Armed with the unusual document, namely, a case history written by me, the patient, Mother went to see the mission doctor and first told him what she knew and how she felt about my circumstances. Following this introductory conversation Mother showed him what I had written about myself. (It was at that point he asked the question about my possible nursing experience.) The doctor then asked Mother to wait whilst he spent a considerable time having a conversation with somebody else and then looking up various books of reference. Mother thought the discussion was with another doctor but she was not sure. Finally, he returned with the name and address of a consultant specialist who, in his opinion, might be able to help. There was no charge for all this time and trouble taken. Looking back on this episode I cannot but marvel as to the kind of help my mother sought and the intuitive feeling she had for doing the right thing. The whole idea was really based on faith, and in this curious way a religious organization was more likely to be sympathetic than the harder, more scientific view held by the old family doctor.

My sister then drafted a letter to this consultant recommended by Dr Rocha, giving my age and specially selected details of my very long and melancholy medical history. Before the letter was posted I well remember my mother and sister coming to see me in hospital and the rather heated discussion which ensued to decide how much to tell the consultant at that stage. It was a delicate situation. Mother was all for telling him as it really was: she said, 'Just tell him the truth – he'll find out in the end, as he will be certain to ask for your hospital notes.' I counselled a certain amount of understatement, since I felt sure he would be entirely put off if he was told all. I became quite belligerent, insisting that a great deal depended on how I looked: in this unaccountable way I looked so much better than I was, I relied on something in the nature of a confidence trick which, oddly enough, actually worked. At the time my mother and sister humoured me and agreed to send a more restrained and modified letter about myself, after which we all awaited his reply with great tenseness. There were two main worries. One was whether he would wish to see me at all, and the other was the delicate question of money and as to how much his fee was likely to be in the event of his agreeing to come. After waiting more than a week, the consultant replied with a guarded letter saying that he would come and see me though he could not promise to be able to do anything (the last few words were underlined) and that the charge would be six guineas. The family breathed a sigh of relief on seeing the fee written down, since guesses as to how much he might charge ranged from ten to twenty-five pounds. To raise the six guineas everything was scraped together from the entire family, including money from my aunt. My sister told me there was also some review as to the manner in which this money was to be paid. It was decided to put the money in an envelope and that Mother would tactfully hand it to the consultant on the day he chose for the visit. All these negotiations took place during the winter months, so that my father was unable to come and see me often or take an active part, since this was the last year of his life. Nevertheless, he was in on all the discussion at home and it was he who raised the question as to how the present ward doctor was to be approached. It was a delicate situation though I certainly did not see it like that at the time, when it was decided to ask me how best he could be told about the impending visit of the specialist. As the ward doctor never made any suggestions regarding my future and usually gave the impression that I did not have one, I blithely thought the entire matter would be of little consequence so far as he was concerned. At the time, there seemed no point in telling the ward doctor anything until there was some definite information as to whether any outside consultant would wish to come and see me at all, so that when Mother asked me what I thought might be the best method of approach to the ward doctor, I cheerfully replied, 'Leave it to me – I will tell him when he comes to do the morning round.' Two days later I broached the subject with the doctor and was quick to notice that he took umbrage at the whole idea. I was left in no doubt that the ward doctor regarded this move as a reflection on the hospital in general and on himself in particular. This was an awkward position. In my eagerness to get things moving, I had reckoned without that subtle matter – medical etiquette. This aspect had simply not crossed my mind. For almost a week the question was left in abeyance. After all, the ward doctor had previously made it quite clear that he was not prepared to do anything, so that he could hardly put up a case to prevent another doctor from making an attempt – even if it was unsuccessful. I dwelt upon the unexpected rebuff I received though it seemed the doctor also had second thoughts, for a few days later he brought the matter up himself. The first reference he made to the suggestion of his own accord was a question weighted with heavy sarcasm. 'Who,' he asked, 'is this world shattering specialist you wish to see?' I gave his name – he was known nationally. The ward doctor said, 'He's much too old!' And continued, 'While your mother was about getting a specialist's opinion, she might have got a younger man – one who would take chances.' At first I was much cast down by this turn of conversation but later decided not to worry. I thought in spite of the assured front they put up to patients it merely proved doctors were human underneath and could even stoop to being sneering and disparaging. There was more to it than that. The well-to-do always had consultations of several specialists if the need arose. It was, however, improper for me to see another doctor. It seemed that medical etiquette operated on two levels. My father sent me a message asking me not to get too involved on the social justice side of the argument because there were double standards for many things and it was possible that the timing of the approach to the ward doctor had been wrong.

Before anything definite happened there were many vicissitudes. The one that worried me most was a letter which the specialist sent to Mother asking her to reconsider the idea of his coming not because he did not want to come, but he had been in touch with this hospital and obtained certain details of my case history. Apparently this information had stiffened his attitude somewhat as he thought it might be a whim on Mother's part, so he asked her to think again and then to phone him. Mother told him she knew enough about my illness to appreciate the serious difficulties, though she would be glad if he would see me, whatever the outcome. So the arrangements were finally concluded and the specialist chose to come on a Saturday morning. I did not know how co-operative the ward doctor would be and was relieved to see both he and Sister were present. In a curious way this gave me moral support.

Sister had made the ward look nice, so that when the specialist walked in, he looked round with some surprise. Although the hospital building was grey and sad, the ward was well kept and cheerful: it compared quite favourably with some voluntary hospitals. Sister's personality had something to do with creating this atmosphere for she was young, good humoured and radiated good health.

The specialist was a very tall man with a walrus moustache; I would have guessed his age as early fifties. His hair was thick, somewhat dishevelled and hung over one side of his forehead in an uncontrolled fringe. He wore a rough tweed suit of cinnamon brown. Moving slowly down the ward towards my bed, they made a rather odd trio. There was the very short, curly-haired ward doctor on one side, in the middle was the very tall, unconventional looking specialist and on the other side walked Sister, red-cheeked, plump and genial. As the trio stopped at my bed, the specialist said 'Hullo' to me rather casually. He stared at me for what seemed a long time and asked, 'How long have you been ill?' I replied, 'Almost four years.' He continued to stare at me and then said rather slowly, 'Nobody would believe it.' I have used the word 'stare' in this context, for that is what the specialist appeared to be doing. He was, in fact, observing me very closely as this kind of observation is as much part of an examination as the physical side. He then took a look at the wound and the cause of all the trouble. His expression changed – he gave a low whistle. The next pause seemed like eternity. I lay there feeling like someone on trial for her life, anxiously awaiting the return of the verdict.

The specialist next said, 'You know I'm not God' – there was another long pause – then he said, 'I will do what I can.' At this point the tension seemed to break and the rest of the conversation continued on a different level. He repeated, 'I cannot promise miracles.' Two or more operations were the least I could expect, for, so far as he could see, I might lie here for another ten years and this would not heal of its own accord. Lastly, addressing myself he said. 'Do you wish to ask me anything?' As I could not think of a question I just thanked him for coming. As he turned to walk out of the ward I heard him say to himself more than anyone else, 'Nothing venture, nothing gain.'

All this time my mother and sister waited outside the ward wondering how the consultation would end. When the specialist came out and told them he would transfer me to his own hospital and there see what he could do for me, a feeling of hope arose though he stressed again that my chances were slim.

Milly was a silent spectator to all this and for a long time she did not comment. During the afternoon she said to me in her direct manner, 'I suppose you are both pleased and frightened.' This really summed up my feelings. I was very pleased as it was a ray of light that some kind of action was contemplated and very frightened because it sounded like a pending Day of Judgment.

So far it had worked according to plan, including my insistence on appearances, though it was Mother who was the prime mover.

From then on started one of the most restless and disturbed periods I ever experienced during this illness. Nobody had mentioned the time factor. I really thought I would move to the other hospital within a week or so, but this was not the case at all – I did not go for months. This waiting seemed so long, that when the ward doctor suggested the other hospital had forgotten about me or, worse still, had changed their minds, I thought it might be true. After waiting for two months the doctor said he would write to the specialist to try and get some information. He did so and the week following I was suddenly told that I would be moving next day. The speed of this decision gave me some anxiety, for I did not know if Mother would get to know in time to accompany me. I was uncertain to the last minute, though it happened to work out well.

I had been in this hospital two years and well remembered the lack of enthusiasm on my arrival. I thought they might be pleased to be rid of me as I was such a lot of work but no, this was not the reaction at all. I concluded that the staff became accustomed to some patients being around for a long time and regarded them as part of the hospital fixtures and fittings. Both staff and patients showed great interest in what was happening to me. Sister, hitherto guarded in her opinions because of the attitude of the ward doctor, now openly gave all the credit to my mother and thought it a good idea for me to have seen an outside doctor for, as she said, he gave my case a fresh, more unbiased look. It made me think again, for I had a lot to learn and took my mother very much for granted. My inner thoughts were really centred on someone else – Milly to be exact. I felt guilty she was being left behind. It bothered me, for I felt she also should have the same chance, though I did not have a clue at the time how all this would end.

On the day of departure from this hospital, I think that Milly was most affected by my going. With her usual self control, however, she did not appear to show it, as she waved me goodbye from the other end of the ward. I had a very friendly send-off from everybody in the ward including the doctor, who by this time had become resigned to the idea of my going.

As I had not seen the outside world for years, I asked the ambulance driver whether he could stop *en route*, so that I might have a look round. He replied it was more than his job was worth to do a thing like that, but he was taking a cut through the park and would drive slowly to enable me to look at the gardens. It was early spring. I well remember how I wished the park was a hundred times bigger so that the ride might last longer. It was a taste of freedom over all too soon, for as the driver came out of the park he speeded up and I soon felt myself going through the gates of the new hospital.

7

I ALWAYS looked round hospital wards in the same way that other people viewed houses or flats. Mentally I asked myself numerous questions. Was the ward cramped or spacious? Was the ward light or shut-in? Were there any extra amenities? What did the general atmosphere feel like? The smell of disinfectant was something all hospitals had in common, otherwise there were differences even in the routine tasks. Having had considerable experience in sizing up different wards I could not assess everything at once, though several things were immediately visible.

The first thing I noticed was the radio and that each bed was fitted with a pair of earphones. Also, there were blue and white cotton check curtains at the side of each bed, which created a semblance of privacy. This ward was on the top floor of the building and very light, with french windows opening out on to a balcony: similar in construction to the very first hospital I was in, where the money for the unemployed young man was collected. The ward contained thirteen beds. In order that the dread number need never be uttered, the thirteenth bed was marked 12A. Here superstition and all manner of inconsistencies bordering on the absurd, went side by side with the last word in scientific discoveries. There was an air of military efficiency which I could not quite place, but discovered afterwards this was linked to tradition. Although by no means one of the oldest hospitals in the country, everyone who worked there behaved as though it was entered in the Domesday Book. But more of this later.

There were three beds empty in the ward and a short discussion took place between the staff and junior nurse, as to which one I was to occupy. The staff nurse was very specific – it seemed I could not be put into any bed.

However, I was totally unprepared for the sensation I encountered following the simple action of being put into bed. Underneath me was the gurgling sound of water. I felt uncomfortably hot, as the water had been warmed to a certain temperature. As I moved in the bed, my body pushed a flow of water to one side. Having never experienced anything like this before, I had some difficulty in working out what type of bed I was in: it then dawned on me I was lying on a full-sized water-pillow, one which covered the entire mattress. All I had previously laid on were air-cushions of varying sizes. Water-pillows were a new experience. These were intended to mitigate against the real misery of soreness caused by lying in bed for long periods. The perpetual movement made me feel uncomfortable. For example, when I tried to sit up, the water travelled down to the bottom of the bed. Although unable to lie on my side, if I turned even slightly the water collected on the opposite side. Neither did the water in the pillow move quietly, for it bubbled and rippled, splashed and cascaded like a miniature Niagara. The idea of the water-pillows was to prevent the body having contact with a hard, rigid surface and thus avoid bedsores. At first, I would have liked to be rid of this water-pillow as the continual movement bothered me, though it was obviously placed there for my especial comfort. And it would be less than fair not to mention the trouble in filling and manipulating those huge rubber pillows, since they took two nurses to hold and place them in position. Nevertheless, I lived on this pillow for months and afterwards became accustomed to the feeling of perpetual movement. When it was finally removed, I felt as though I had fallen out of the water on to the rocks.

Some time later the ward sister came to look me over. She was a woman in the late forties, of medium height, a fresh complexion and rather fuzzy hair. With a ready laugh she exclaimed, 'Why I thought you were about ten years old!' 'Ten years old,' I repeated with scorn, 'I'm twice that age.' (The specialist had told Sister he was having a child brought into the ward who would have to stay for a long time and for whom he felt sorry. With clear diction, a good command of language and great authority, Sister had the voice and manner of one accustomed to giving orders.

This, my first encounter with Sister, showed her at her best.

Actually she was formidable. Judging by age she must have started her training at the turn of the century and was one of the martinet type that have since become almost extinct. An excellent nurse, a good organizer and teacher – the ward was run like clockwork. However, it was very much a one-party system and there was no opposition.

Sister had no respect whatsoever for people under her charge. Those included were nurses, patients and all their relations, medical students and ward cleaners. She regarded house surgeons as semi-respectable and spoke to them with a certain condescension and some contempt. Her attitude towards almoners was on a somewhat higher level, since their co-operation might sometimes prove useful. In ordinary speech Sister was fond of the use of the imperative and would say, 'Go' or 'Come' or 'Speak'. Completely unpredictable, she was a curious mixture of Florence Nightingale and Boadicea. Months later the following conversation took place between the night nurse and one of the house surgeons on night duty. The doctor said, 'Sister H. has a very dominating personality', to which the night nurse swiftly replied, 'You mean domineering.'

There was a great deal of activity on this ward—during the daytime it was hardly ever free of doctors or medical students. The doctors were around at mealtimes, visiting times and late at night. It was not unusual for the specialist to come and see me at 10 p.m. Sister could not say anything to the doctors when they arrived at odd hours, but she could to the medical students and they received the full brunt of her temper. The students were allowed in at certain times and had to ask Sister's permission to enter the ward. She rarely refused permission but rationed their time. They would politely knock and ask Sister, 'Is it all right to come into the ward.' She would reply, 'Yes, until twelve noon only and not a minute after.' This was literally true for, on the stroke of twelve if they were not on their way out, she would inquire with crushing sarcasm, 'Can't you tell the time?' The students breathed a sigh of relief if Sister was off duty, for their association with the nurses was on quite a different level.

The patient was never consulted on the question of the use of students, if the doctor thought the illness of any patient might be of teaching interest. Sometimes the patient would be admitted into hospital with one illness, and used for demonstration purposes for something totally different as, for example, in the following instance. There was a young woman in the ward with uncomplicated appendix trouble – what the Staff called a 'clean appendix'. She happened to have a club-foot, so this was made the subject of a teaching demonstration for a large class of students. She was not told what was going to happen: the consultant, followed by a crowd of students, descended on her quite suddenly and completely surrounded her bed. The young woman was extremely agitated about the way in which she was used, though all her complaints were made to the other patients in strict privacy.

Usually one or two students were allocated to each patient. They asked much the same questions as the doctor had asked previously and learned to take down case histories.

This was followed by a general examination, during which the student was careful not to utter any kind of opinion. Afterwards the doctor might question the student on his findings and the reasons for his conclusions. This form of cross-questioning sometimes took place near the patient's bedside, though some of the groups moved and continued discussions well out of range of the patient's hearing. I never became accustomed to the curious feeling when the entire conversation would be about myself and yet I was in no way part of it, or seemingly remotely connected. I might just as well have been a corpse or a fictional case as a live one. Yet there was no mistaking the fact that the conversation was about a living, human being – me! The very large classes of students were frightening. Headed by the consultant, they used to tramp through the ward like an army and use the patient as an inanimate object. Some patients said this did not bother them. However, when the ward was at last free, there was no mistaking the sense of relief – even by those who were apparently not bothered. If the truth were known, I expect the students were much more afraid of the patient than vice versa.

So far as the patients were concerned, the students were well behaved and most, very considerate. They would often do small favours for us such as handing things out of lockers, or leaving drinks and other necessaries within reach. (If all this does not sound very significant, I hasten to stress its importance. Patients who cannot move or help themselves have the awful feeling of being partly or wholly dependent on others. It creates great frustration having to ask for all those things to be done, which in the ordinary way, people do for themselves automatically, such as sitting up or reaching for a glass of water and a host of other things.)

There have been changes with regard to the use of medical students in teaching hospitals. The patient now has the right of refusal. This right is not often exercised mainly because the law is difficult to implement, since the students are often upon the patient before he or she has time to say 'No', although the polite phrase 'do you mind', is always quietly spoken by somebody. Another difficulty, moreover, is that the patient is often a captive partner. On the subject of medical students, I once heard an amusing exchange between a patient and the doctor. She asked the doctor whether a certain clinic (and here she named one of the largest and most expensive private clinics in the country) had medical students. The doctor was very quick and answered, 'Certainly not, it is not a recognized training school.'

Patients are people. Most people appreciate the fact that new doctors have to be trained and there is no other way of training except by the present methods. It is the 'bull in the china shop' approach that creates resentment. A modicum of tact and understanding soon dispels the patient's feeling of affront, which is mostly based on fear.

Coloured students at this hospital were completely segregated. They formed a group of their own and occasionally did a special round with one of the hospital consultants. If the coloured students were segregated, women students and doctors were ostracized. Women were being trained at the Royal Free and Elizabeth Garret Anderson hospitals, though there were no women in this hospital. Neither were they admitted into the majority of other voluntary hospitals that were recognized training schools.

The term 'restrictive practices' is much used in connection with industry. This conception is not new and has been used in many other ways other than labour struggles. During the 1914–18 war, women students were admitted to all London training hospitals and women doctors used in many fields of medicine. As soon as the first world war ended the intake of women medical students started to slow down. Thus, in 1931, when I came to this hospital, which was one of the well-known training schools, there were no women students or doctors.

The move to the present hospital made a great difference to me because of the excellent treatment. This was very important since it helped to lessen the pain. After a few days the specialist came to see me and said that he would not give special instructions about dressings, but he expected Sister to see to it that I was never uncomfortable. Sister dutifully replied, 'Yes, sir,' and faithfully carried out the order. However, she was fond of telling me I was a great expense to the hospital, as I cost about three pounds a week in dressings.

Having no idea of what was going to happen to me, I was always apprehensive when the specialist came. The next time he came to see me I was surprised to hear him say to Sister, 'You know she has been in hospital such a long time, she must have a change of air.' He went on to stress that he was not prepared to do anything until I had this break. This posed a problem. Sister became really alarmed and started to explain that there were no places equipped to take anyone like myself, since I needed too much attention. Before Sister could finish this explanation, the specialist held up his hand in the manner of a policeman on point duty stopping the traffic and said, 'Sister, I am not interested in hearing about the difficulties, you must explore every possibility'. As I watched him disappear through the ward door resplendent in his cinnamon coloured suit, I felt caught between the upper and nether millstones of his commands and the irritation of Sister.

Sister regarded all this as totally unreasonable, though she had to do something. Next day she enlisted the help of the house surgeon and he commiserated, both agreeing it was a difficult situation. The house surgeon promised to make some inquiries; Sister would get in touch with the almoner, and between them try and work out something. Two weeks later I was no nearer going convalescent. The specialist came again and said, 'Are you still here?' This was self-evident. Sister explained there were serious difficulties in trying to get me away. He listened without interrupting and when she had finished speaking quietly said, 'Sister, when I come again I do not expect to find her still here.' (He was, of course, referring to myself.) Being a tall man he covered ground quickly and seemed to be out of the ward before Sister had time to rally. Then, as now, an instruction from a consultant was like the law of the Medes and Persians. Compared to the lamentations of Sister, Jeremiah appeared uncomplaining. It really was an awkward situation. The following week the house surgeon, the almoner and Sister between them managed to get me away for a couple of weeks. At first, I wondered how this feat was accomplished. However, a short time later, certain aspects of this combined operation became much clearer.

In most hospitals patients were told as little as possible and more especially in this one, so that I was mildly surprised when the house surgeon took the trouble to read me the letter he proposed sending to the matron of the convalescent home which had agreed to take me. The purpose of this letter was to give the impression that I was much better than was actually the case, and the object in reading me the content was for me to play my part in maintaining that impression. I got the message.

The journey to this convalescent home was a nightmare. I had to go most of the way by train and recall having to lie on the seat of the compartment as there was no other way of getting off my feet. A car met me at the other end and I arrived thoroughly exhausted. As Sister quite rightly pointed out, those places were not equipped to care for people such as myself. Along with the change of air I also had a great deal of trouble. The convalescent doctor was distinctly annoyed with the hospital for sending me, and during the first week there was talk of returning me to the hospital. I found the whole episode upsetting. If the idea was to get me down there and trust to luck that the convalescent matron would make allowances and not refuse to keep me, it worked quite well. I certainly did my share by trying to pretend there were no difficulties, though the convalescent staff quite openly said that 'the hospital had pulled a fast one on them', which indeed they had. I was also very lonely as most of the other people were able to get out and about. For most part of the day I spent hours in bed without seeing anybody, except when someone remembered the dressing needed changing, etc. The weather was very good, so that in spite of the difficulties I began to look a better colour and by the end of the two weeks, all agreed my general condition had improved.

Although the convalescent staff were kind to me, especially the doctor, they were relieved when I left, for I was a strain on their staff and resources. I made the return journey the same way I had come and was glad to return to the ward. I was surprised how few of the ward patients I knew, since most had gone home during the time I was away.

The orders about my going convalescent had been carried out – the staff were in the clear. I improved in spite of the *ad hoc* arrangements, not because of them.

On my return to the hospital there was a pretty girl in the next bed who told me she had some form of heart trouble. It seemed she was an only child aged nineteen and her parents made every effort for her to see any consultant who might suggest something to help her. She was accustomed to being in hospital. In reply to my question 'Have you been here long?' she replied, 'Only two days.' She added that Sister had told her she would be moving to another ward. Heart disease in all its forms was regarded as 'medical', so that I was surprised she was in this ward which was designated as 'surgical'. A few minutes after this conversation three doctors came into the ward and approached the girl with the heart complaint. The curtains were drawn round her bed, so that she was invisible to the rest of us. However, I noticed one of the doctors holding what appeared to be a large jam jar, full of water and in the jar was a creature which resembled a dark coloured worm about three inches long. I had no idea what this was about. Sister, of course, was present and apart from a certain amount of moving around behind the curtains, all was quiet. A short time passed and the doctors emerged from behind the curtains, one still carrying the jar containing the worm, which seemed to me much larger than at first glance. He held the jar behind his back and had a short discussion with the other two doctors away from the girl's bed. I could not hear any of the conversation. After this all three left the ward, the doctor still holding the jar as though he was trying to render it invisible.

Following the exit of the three doctors, Sister called all the ward nurses together and gave a short dissertation on what had just happened. 'Why?' asked Sister, 'should the doctor want to draw blood from a girl who is already very anaemic?' If any of the nurses knew the answer they were not quick enough, for Sister continued by answering her own question, 'Because the blood is flowing in the wrong channels.' I do not remember the rest of the conversation, or it might even have ended at this point.

Later I asked the young girl in the next bed, who looked more dead than alive, what had been happening. She did not know, except that she felt absolutely awful, although she had no pain. Still pondering, I said, 'I wonder what that creature was in the jar?' Neither of us knew. Curiosity got the better of me, so I later repeated the question to the junior nurse serving the suppers. 'Nurse, what was that little creature in the jar?' The junior nurse replied briskly, 'You were not supposed to be looking.' I pressed on, 'Do you mean to say I will die without ever knowing?' 'You're not in imminent danger of death – I might tell you about it afterwards.' Nurse was as good as her word. When she came to tidy the beds for the night she started the conversation herself with, 'In case you die of curiosity that creature the doctor carried around in the jar was – a leech.'

At his next visit following my return to the ward, the specialist beamed with pleasure and thought I looked much better. He then turned to Sister and said, 'Well done.' She positively purred with delight and replied, 'Not at all, sir.' Following this round of congratulations, the specialist cheerfully announced that he was going on holiday for a few weeks and would decide what to do on his return. Circulating in my mind was the thought, 'I have been in hospital for years, so what difference will a few weeks make?'

I have already commented on the unconventional clothes worn by the specialist when he first came to see me. I never saw him wear anything different than a cinnamon coloured suit, made from heavy tweed. I decided his tailor must have had an unlimited supply of this tweed and that from time to time, he merely ordered a repeat of the previous suit.

The entire situation fascinated me because his outfits were diametrically opposed to the general tone of the hospital. All the other consultants appeared on the ward wearing black jackets and striped trousers. Occasionally they would come wearing long, white coats. I could scarcely believe my eyes when I first noticed these were not merely white coats – but, white coats with tails! Most things worn or used in this hospital had little to do with comfort or convenience – it was all geared to tradition.

The chairman of this hospital was a noble Lord. Famous for his fund-raising schemes and very deaf. I remember him coming into the ward one afternoon. It was an 'Open Day', when the Governors and all who donated to the upkeep of the hospital walked round the wards, speaking to patients if they felt so inclined. We had all previously been briefed by Sister in the following way. We were to speak only when directly addressed: we were not to give detailed descriptions about illness. (Milly would have thoroughly approved.) And finally, she (Sister) hoped that nobody would complain about anything for, 'As we were all aware, there was nothing whatsoever to complain about.' As a matter of fact, an elderly Dowager asked me about the food – did I enjoy it? Remembering Sister's order of the day, I hastened to reply, 'It is delicious.'

The noble Lord's function as hospital chairman was mainly concerned with plans for raising money to keep the hospital going – which was no easy matter. Huge notices were displayed in the foreground, informing all who wished to read about the financial plight of the hospital. At intervals, certain wards would temporarily close in order to economize. In this manner the hospital staggered from crisis to crisis. Of course, certain basic minima were guaranteed by moneys left in wills, income from property, ward and bed endowments and payments made by patients. But this was never sufficient to cover the hospital needs or make expansion possible, without further debt being incurred.

It was also interesting to note the almost dictatorial power exercised by the chairman. Among other accomplishments he was, no doubt, very able at raising money for the hospital, though his ideas in other ways were somewhat rigid. For example, it was open talk among the nurses that he refused to accept girls for nursing training who had their hair cut short. Short hair for women had become very fashionable. It seemed the chairman disliked this fashion and acted accordingly. In the war against fashion he was finally beaten and had to capitulate, for his insistence on nurses having long hair, created a shortage.

One day, the ward radio, usually rather feeble, was tuned in to its fullest capacity. The sound volume was centrally controlled and none of the patients knew why it was tuned in so loud. All headphones had to be disconnected as the noise was shattering. Next day one of the nurses told me that the hospital chairman was ill and as he was hard of hearing, Matron decided to turn the radio on full blast for his benefit. I believe it was a fatal illness though, at the time, no one in the ward had the faintest idea of what was happening.

I used to amuse myself by trying to remember all the different kinds of uniforms I had seen nurses wear: these varied in design and colour in each hospital. Some nurses wore pink and white striped uniforms; others blue and white stripes. There were also plain uniforms in colours of blue or lilac and many other types. Nurses wore different coloured uniforms within the same hospital, to denote different grades. Waistbelts varied, as did the white top-aprons. Some aprons had bibs attached to the top of the uniform by two pins, others had bands which went over the shoulders and fastened at the back. Many of the uniforms included ghastly stiff, white starched collars and cuffs, which were hot and troublesome, because they chafed the skin. Outdoor uniforms differed, some wore coats, others full-length capes. The short, red-lined capes for nurses intended as casual wear, were introduced about 1930. Prior to this I recall nurses wearing their own woollen jackets and cardigans. The exception to the formal uniforms were the nurses from religious orders, who wore their own habit; again in different colours such as white, brown or cream nun's veiling.

The uniform worn by nurses in this hospital was sensible and comfortable if old fashioned, since their skirts had to be the regulation eight inches from the ground. It was the caps that formed part of the sisters' uniform which were strange and obsolete. These were very elaborate and hung down to the waistline at the back in a long, pleated panel; the long back panel caught on door handles, corners or anything else that happened to be in the way.

One day, when Sister's cap was almost wrenched off her head because the piece that hung down at the back had caught between the ward doors, I mildly remarked that the cap seemed somewhat inconvenient. Having spoken out of turn, Sister approached my bed, purple in the face with indignation, as she hastily pinned her cap back into position, and asked threateningly, 'Do you recommend that the design of the caps be altered?' I tentatively suggested, 'Perhaps the cap could be modified.' I considered this to be a mild understatement though Sister became even more angry with me and said, 'Do you realize, girl, this cap and uniform was designed by a famous matron of this hospital and that the late Queen took an interest!' On receiving this news I was reduced to silence: privately I thought the design of the caps very odd.

When I was young I was obliged to attend laundry classes, as it was then considered to be an integral part of my education. There I learned how to wash and iron clothes, how to scrub tables and, among other things, how to use goffering irons. To people who have never seen goffering irons they are best described as a type of curling iron, similar to those once used in hairdressing. The goffering irons were heated over an open flame and used for ironing short pleats. Each pleat had to be done separately. I record this to give some idea as to the amount of work involved in laundering the sisters' caps, as these contained yards of this type of pleating, consisting of scores of individual pleats. I used to think it very strange at the time. The hospital finances were in a permanent state of precariousness, yet in order to maintain an outmoded, useless fashion, which was really a whim, wages would have to be paid to those employed in the hospital laundry for the purpose of goffering the caps. Of course, work of such nature was only possible because labour was very cheap.

While writing about the sisters' caps, forty years on, my thoughts returned to the strange things about the hospital, which were always impressed on me as the great hospital tradition. Knowing that goffering irons have become museum pieces, I wondered whether the caps had been relegated to stage props. However, looking back on the powerful hospital tradition, the more I thought about it, the less sure I became of what did happen to the sisters' caps. A startling thought entered my head. Was it possible they still wore them? I dwelt on this aspect and finally decided to visit the hospital to find out the fate of the caps. I went to the hospital laundry.

I remembered exactly where the laundry was sited at the back of the hospital, because one of the balconies in the ward which I was in gave a clear, uninterrupted view of the place. In fact, it was visible for miles around as it had a very tall, brick-built chimney which, in the days before skyscrapers, towered above all the surrounding buildings. I spent a fascinating hour in the hospital laundry but, before entering, I had a good look outside. Forty years later, in spite of the tall, new blocks built all around – the brick chimney still maintained its dominating position.

The first person I met was an older woman, who told me she was a supervisor and had worked in the laundry for years. When I confided in her the purpose of my visit, she was most interested and co-operative. She explained to me that the sisters' uniforms had been changed and they no longer wore the caps with the long panels. But, the supervisor went on to tell me, on special occasions such as nurses' graduation or prize giving, the sisters wore the clothes I remembered. They were now worn as a dress uniform for special occasions. I then asked how the caps were laundered. In these days, I supposed the sisters' caps were made to a modern method of permanent pleating, so imagine my amazement when the supervisor replied, 'With goffering irons, we still use the old method – would you like to see them?' She led me upstairs to the next floor. As I followed her into a very large room, I felt I had stepped back two whole eras – into the Edwardian and Victorian worlds.

In this room I saw a number of women busily engaged in ironing by hand. My attention was drawn to a large bench, upon which stood a quaint gas apparatus – used for goffering. This gas apparatus was contained in a three-sided, black iron canopy, with the gas piping built into the wall. On top was a grid with a large spread flame, similar to that of an eye-level grill or toaster in a modern gas stove. Above the gas jets were deep holes, into which several pairs of goffering irons could be inserted and heated at the same time. A few pairs of goffering irons were lying on the bench. I noticed that the scissor-like handles of these had been bound with muslin, to increase the grip of the fingers and prevent slipping. Tradition certainly dies hard. On my way home from the hospital laundry I wondered what Milly would have said with her laconic, penetrating comments, about the visit, the caps and the goffering irons.

I must now go back and continue my story which came to a temporary halt, because the specialist went away on holiday for over a month.

Having returned from his holiday the specialist came into the ward to see me quite late one night. I was asleep and he did not wake me. I hardly ever slept more than an hour at a time. Being in bed day and night had a curious effect on my sleep rhythm. I used to fall asleep for short periods and keep waking up, because of the noise in the ward and the nagging pain. When I awoke the night nurse told me about this visit and I naturally asked, 'What did the doctor say?' Nurse replied somewhat guardedly, 'Oh, the day staff will tell you all about it.' There was a sharp line of demarcation between the duties and responsibilities of the night and day staffs. Obviously, the specialist had made a definite statement of some kind; the night nurse would not tell me, as it was not within her sphere of duty to give me this information. In fact, I did not know what had been said until the afternoon of the following day. It was then that Sister suddenly said, 'Number six, you are for operation on Wednesday.' Here I must explain Sister's odd habit of calling patients by the number of the bed which they happened to occupy. After some time patients became accustomed to this mode of address, though it was not very endearing. It was reminiscent of army methods and I do not recall this type of approach in any other hospital. Later, when I had been in the ward longer than anyone else, I was asked more than once whether I still remembered my proper name, since it was rarely used other than visiting times.

I was pleased to be told of this pending operation at very short notice – it gave me less time to dwell upon it. I remembered the specialist telling me that two operations were the least I could expect and I rightly deduced this coming operation would be exploratory. Although I was X-rayed many times during the period I was ill, I had a condition which did not show on an X-ray plate.

People react very differently towards operations. Some patients told me they experienced no feelings of fear or panic either before or after an operation. Alternatively, I have seen people react violently to surgery considered to be slight. From my own experience, the conflict of emotions made it difficult to be objective. Consciousness and semi-consciousness, reality and unreality, shock, fear and relief, all form part of the pattern of reaction. I had the dual feeling of both wanting the operation since I knew it could not be avoided and of being afraid of what might happen.

Following this operation I suffered rather less from the after-effects of the anaesthetic, possibly because I did not have so much, as I was told it was of relatively short duration. (Others in the ward always kept a time check as to when patients went from the ward and returned.) It was exploratory and little was done in actual surgery. Yet, this was one of the most painful and uncomfortable operations I ever experienced. The healing process was very slow and the intense soreness continued for weeks. Some pain is not serious in the sense that it is symptomatic of deep-rooted causes, yet can be nerve fraying, wearing and extremely lowering by its very persistence. However, as nothing was done to try and lessen the pain, it had to be endured. The attitude towards pain had changed little over the years I was ill. If anything, this hospital was case-hardened to a point of callousness. The doctor in the council hospital who put me on a drug, in spite of the after-effects, was ahead of his time in medical thinking.

Many methods used in this ward were old fashioned, compared even to the council hospital from which I had just come. A good illustration were the trolleys used for dressings. These were actually tiled tables on wheels, with a lower shelf, also tiled. It seemed hard to believe these trolleys were purpose designed, because there was no rim or guard round the edges. With monotonous regularity bowls and instruments in use on the tables, fell over the edge. All dishes and bowls were then made of enamel, not from stainless steel as they are today, so there was not only a clatter, but the enamel chipped. A similar situation applied to the medicine round, for which these trolleys were also used. As nearly all medicines were in liquid form at that time, the nurse in charge kept a wary eye on the trolley. In spite of this, many a bottle worked its way over the edge and ended with a crash on the floor. Mopping up was a fairly constant procedure. Moreover, the trolleys were very low and many of the nurses had to stoop quite sharply in order to push them round the ward. The hospital was very large and where a change of equipment involved all wards, it may have been a question of money. It might also have been a question of attitude for, as with the sisters' caps, even if life was made more difficult by retaining old-established methods and fashions, the very thought of a break with traditional usage created stiff resistance in the people responsible for top administration.

Although it was difficult to equate the tense feeling in this ward with gaiety, as well as the radio, the ward also boasted of a gramophone. This gramophone was of the nineteen-twenty vintage with a huge horn and powerful winding handle and on one side was a brass plate, giving the name of the person by whom it had been donated. It was played only very occasionally. I wonder really it was ever played at all, since to do this required a rare combination of circumstances. Obviously, the gramophone could not be played if anyone in the ward was very ill. Neither could it be played if a doctor or others of importance were in the ward. Sister never allowed it to be played while she was on duty, for she regarded such a pastime as frivolous, trivial and non-essential. The gramophone was rather difficult to manipulate as it needed a great deal of winding and this, in turn, meant that the person who played it had to feel relatively well. As a matter of fact it was always played by the younger patients when they were getting better. I always made it my business to tell other patients there was a gramophone around, as it was housed in one of the numerous cupboards outside the ward. The nurses were very obliging and would always carry it in on the rare occasions it was played, for although the horn and winding handle were detachable, it was very heavy. There usually followed a short conference to decide where the gramophone should be placed as, complete with horn and winding handle, it took up considerable space. The best place to deposit it was on someone's bed table so that the horn could be positioned across the bed, making it relatively unobtrusive.

The gramophone recitals were usually short-lived: neither did they end very gracefully. The fact that the gramophone was loud also made things difficult, as it seemed impossible to reduce or control the sound. It started off with a vibrating blast, which gave some of the patients a shock. I did try to prepare them for this beforehand by saying, 'Well, the gramophone is all right but it's rather loud.' Sometimes the needle would stick in the groove of the record and the tune would repeat itself over and over again. The needle would then have to be pushed forward slightly, so that the tune might continue. The repertoire consisted of about ten records which were either marches or waltz tunes, so that the choice was limited. After a while somebody would invariably say, 'We've heard that one before.' It nearly always ended with someone complaining of a headache and, whilst there was no direct accusation that the gramophone was responsible, it was put away until another opportunity presented itself.

Sometimes the frustration of lying in bed would come upon me so forcibly that I really felt something awful would happen if I did not get up. This feeling was connected with playing the gramophone one summer afternoon. There were several young people in the ward, up and about, on the verge of going home. They decided to try dancing: needless to say it was Sister's week-end off. I loved dancing and was with them in spirit as I followed the dancers round with my eyes, though it took me a couple of days to fight off the irritation, which was like a state of agitated excitability.

I commented earlier on the different atmosphere in hospital wards and thought it hard to give exact reasons for this. To a great extent the tone is set by the sister. The nurses change but the sister remains. Nurses would often judge a ward or department by the sister in charge and what she was like to work for. There was a strained atmosphere in this ward. When Sister was off duty or on holiday, the entire ward relaxed – patients and staff. One week-end when Sister was away and the ward rather less hectic than usual, I thought on other things and came to the conclusion that I fancied chipped potatoes. Unlike the present time, I cannot ever recall having chips in hospital. It was probably their association with the unhygienic, steamy fish and chip shops of the time, when chips for 'taking away' were doused with vinegar and wrapped in newspaper. Chips were not then elevated to the exalted position they now hold as 'French Fried'. To request such a dish would not have entered my head. It was merely that I made the observation during the evening bed-making session, when a generalized conversation about food was in progress. When nurse finished making the beds, she disappeared into the kitchen and, to my great astonishment, later emerged with a plate of chips for me. Handing me the chips nurse said, 'Here you are, my dear, it did not seem much to ask for.' To say that such an act would have been unthinkable had Sister been on duty, is really a masterpiece of understatement. It was also an example and tribute to what nurses often did for patients quite outside their ordinary duties.

Sister's attitude towards the nurses was sometimes worse than the way she behaved to patients. There was certainly no privileged class among those she considered 'the lower orders'. Nearly all the nurses were young and many very attractive. One afternoon the staff nurse returned to the ward after her off-duty period with slight make-up on her face. Sister pounced on her immediately and in a voice audible right across the ward said, 'Nurse, how dare you come on duty with that stuff on your face – go and wash it off at once!'

Staff nurse flushed very red and left the ward; when she returned we could see she had been crying. To so humiliate another member of the staff as to make her the cynosure of all eyes was part of the power of the ward sister, and her intolerable interference with personal liberty was taken for granted.

Occasionally Sister's unpredictable attitude might show itself in other and kinder ways, such as the following.

My young brother, still at school, used to come and see me at the normal visiting times. One day Sister told him he might also come to see me on Tuesday between seven and eight in the evening. The suddenness of this gesture took us both by surprise. For the next four months my young brother came to see me every Tuesday evening – an extra visiting hour was a great privilege. We were very fond of each other and I always looked forward to his coming. Just as suddenly, one day Sister told him not to come any more, except on Sundays and Wednesdays at the usual visiting hours. It was a great disappointment when he stopped coming, as I had become accustomed to seeing him each Tuesday. No one had the temerity to question Sister's authority – she was a law unto herself.

Side by side with Sister's dictatorial approach based on personal whims, she also had a sizeable following among the other ward sisters. On alternate Thursdays she arranged her off-duty period in the afternoon, when quite a procession of sisters from other wards would come and take tea with her. The patients used to watch the sisters with great interest since they had to walk right through the ward, on their way to the tea party. Also, Sister gave the ward-maid (whom she bullied unmercifully) explicit instructions as to how many were expected to tea in her room. Sister had her own room at the far end of the ward. I am unable to describe this room to the reader, for I never ever looked at it from the inside. The nearest I came to seeing it was one day just before I left hospital, the door was slightly ajar and I noticed two china ornaments standing on an unidentifiable piece of furniture. It was as though an invisible, armed sentry guarded the entrance to Sister's room and no ordinary mortal was allowed to see inside. There have been all kinds of tea parties, real and fictional. Alas, there are no records of real tea parties, only fictional ones such as the 'not bloody likely' one in Shaw's *Pygmalion*, or the Mad Hatter's tea party in *Alice in Wonderland*. I often wondered what Sister's tea parties were like and what topics were discussed.

The never-ending cycle of ward work went on every day and most of the night. There were also many tasks little to do with nursing performed at less regular intervals. One of these was changing the blue check bed curtains and cleaning the iron supports on which the curtains hung. This was done at roughly three-monthly intervals when the nurses were less busy.

At such a period of curtain changing, one of the young patients came over to have a chat with me; she confided that she felt very depressed. I sympathized and commiserated with her, though it was obvious she was in a low state of deep depression. This girl was only seventeen and had what was thought to be arthritis in both hips: she walked with great difficulty. In the course of this conversation one of the things she said was, 'I feel I could run away from here.' This being quite a common reaction in hospital, I did not pay particular attention to this remark. A while later Sister told the girl to go downstairs and sit in the hospital grounds to get some fresh air, as the weather was fine. She borrowed something to read from me and limped out of the ward on her way to the lift. That was the last we saw of her.

The girl went downstairs after tea at about three-thirty in the afternoon – she was not missed until the evening meal at six o'clock. It seemed she walked out of the gate at the back of the hospital grounds and somehow reached her home without arousing too much curiosity, considering she was in her dressing-gown. Sister had been off-duty. She returned to the ward as the alarm was raised that the girl was missing. The short conversation she had with me proved most unfortunate. Sister was very suspicious at the best of times. She now became firmly convinced I was implicated in a deep conspiracy with this girl. The police were informed and naturally went first to her home where she was found unharmed, but determined not to return to the hospital. That was certainly not the end of the matter so far as I was concerned. Before she went down to the hospital grounds, Sister remembered the girl and myself were engaged in conversation. I was, therefore, commanded by Sister to repeat every word of that conversation. The entire episode took on a criminal aspect.

Sister approached me in the usual overbearing manner she reserved for patients and said, 'Are you aware that number three has run away?' I replied, 'I heard from Nurse she did not return from the garden.' Sister continued threateningly, 'I want you to tell me every word she said to you.' I told what I recalled of the conversation. When I repeated the words 'She was very depressed and felt she could run away,' Sister stared at me in amazement and shouted, 'Do you mean to tell me she said a thing like that and you did not tell anybody?' I informed Sister it was not unusual for patients to say things like that and I had often heard those words. (I had said this myself to other patients many times, though thought it best not to mention the fact.) Sister could scarcely believe her ears when she heard those words were not original and had been uttered before. She continued to declaim to the ward patients in general and myself in particular. 'Number three, an ungrateful and selfish patient had given everyone a great deal of trouble – the doctor had taken her into hospital to see what could be done for her and instead of being thankful – she had run away'. Sister felt personally affronted and outraged. No doubt she also had to give a detailed account of what happened to her superiors.

On the question of depression. So far as I was concerned and I think I was fairly typical, I would not have dreamed of telling the doctor or any other member of the staff that I felt depressed, since it would not have been regarded as a relevant symptom. Of course depression existed, but it was an abstraction. Patients might mention it to each other in the way that the girl who ran away from the ward mentioned it to me, though it would go no further. One either had pain or did not have pain. There had to be a visible or recognized symptom. To illustrate the point. One of the ward patients had a blood transfusion. These were given at great risk because the different blood groups were not then known. The woman later complained she felt ill. Sister said she should feel better and only imagined she was ill because of the transfusion. As the day went on the woman became progressively more ill and said she had severe pain. Sister started to take notice only when it was discovered she ran a high temperature. Once a tangible symptom appeared Sister took note and thought it appropriate to inform the doctor. When I was in the previous council hospital I became very low-spirited following the unexpected failure of an operation which I was led to expect held no great risk. The doctor told Sister one morning I was being histrionic. Depression was totally disregarded in all the different wards I was in.

Perhaps the story just told might be regarded as unconnected with the story I am about to tell. There is a connection – it lies in the way people behave under great stress. The young girl in the ward having reached a point at which she could not cope, ran out of the hospital clad in her dressing gown. The woman in the story that follows also ran out of the hospital – though under different circumstances. The fact that the next story happened not in this hospital but in the street, when I was nine years old, in no way dims my memory. It was unforgettable.

One hot, summer afternoon, my sister, myself and a mutual friend found ourselves bored. (Our combined age was under thirty.) Children often suffer from boredom and we were no exception. There was nothing better to do so we decided to walk along the main road. We had no particular destination. Having walked about a quarter of a mile a woman approached us and asked the way to a place the other side of the district. Because it was near our school we children all knew this place and, speaking together, told her it was too far to walk and she would have to ride. The woman had a strange look on her face. Even more strange, however, was the large bundle she carried in her arms. She was carrying something wrapped up in a large top coat. We children stared at this bundle for at one end there were curls hanging out – the curls of human hair. When the woman heard what we said about having to ride where she wanted to go, she stood staring into space. Suddenly she turned and, facing us, said 'Are you looking at what I'm carrying? It's my little boy – he's dead. I just brought him out of hospital – I don't want *them* to bury him – *I* want him home.' With those words, she hoisted the bundle containing the dead child more firmly in her arms and walked away from us.

Next time the specialist came to see me he did not speak, but looked at me for what seemed a long time – then gave a long, drawn-out sigh. I found sighs very difficult to interpret as they can be associated with boredom, irritability, condolence or resignation, etc. I could not tell from the tone of the sigh to which group it belonged for, like all doctors, he was trained to give away nothing he did not wish to tell. Despite the fact that the specialist was rather testy and a trifle eccentric, I liked him because he was free of cant and hypocrisy and not without a sense of humour.

Following the sigh he said to me in his rather sad fashion, 'You are more worry to me than all my money.' I did not reply. Privately I thought, 'You can pay someone to look after your money, though it would be less easy to find anybody to whom the responsibility of myself could be passed on.' I really believed he was just as afraid of me as I was of him – for different reasons. The last operation I had was painful and uncomfortable, but fairly superficial. My guess was that it did not give the specialist much more information than he already knew. He would have to take a chance with me: without anything definite being said I could tell he was making up his mind not what to do, but when to do it. There was to be a real showdown in the sense that he staked his experience as a surgeon against the failure of previous surgeons. It was a challenge. As he had already made his name as a famous surgeon it seemed to me there could only be one loser – myself. Looking back it was hardly fair to think that way, since he need not have taken me on at all. He was a compassionate man and also courageous, for I was an unknown quantity. No decision was taken, so I continued in the ward with the situation hanging fire as it were.

However much I tried, I could not get away from the drama and tragedy that was part of my everyday life. I remembered the notice Milly had on her bed-table, informing all that she did not wish to discuss illness. Events often spoke for themselves – one did not have to discuss them. Of the many illustrations I could give I have chosen two; the first for its tragedy and the second for its pathos.

Mrs Hochsten, pale, dark-haired, with very bright eyes, was a relatively young woman. Accompanied by her two teenage daughters she had come from South Africa to see a specialist in this hospital, as she had a tumour on the spine. I recall the doctor asking her unusual questions, such as what she took against malaria, so that the same tablets could be ordered for her to maintain regular routine. Unable to walk, she was in the ward for some weeks before an operation was finally attempted. The operation lasted so long, most of us thought the worst and that she would not return. Quite late in the evening she was returned to the ward, having been away for nine hours. From then on started a four weeks' struggle to try and save her life. This fight literally continued by day and by night but to no avail – it ended in her death. It was a drama in which we were all involved: the medical staff, the nursing staff, together with all the patients in the ward. On the days when Mrs Hochsten was better, there was a relaxation of tension in the entire ward. During those four weeks she was close to death many times yet, with the help of the staff who always hovered round her and the tremendous fight for life she herself put up, somehow she managed to rally and live another day. Had the same thing happened at the present time, Mrs Hochsten would have been in an intensive care unit. At that time there was not even a side-room for anybody so desperately ill and, like many others, she lived and died in public. In this ward it was the curtains round the bed and in other hospitals merely the screens, that separated the living, the dying and the dead. Her two daughters showed tremendous faith and were convinced their mother would recover and all three would return home to South Africa. This was not to be, the two sisters went home without their mother. We in the ward, who watched this four-week drama hour by hour, were much affected by all that happened; although only onlookers we were all emotionally highly involved. I was reminded of the words of John Donne, 'When any man dies I am diminished, for am I not one of mankind . . .'

The next story was one of the most pathetic I have ever witnessed, yet it took place with hardly a word spoken. In an effort to capture an experience, I have often read long descriptions and dialogue. It is possible to transmit the most intense feelings without action and without words. There is a form of silent communication so powerful that none could mistake its meaning.

There was a very old lady in the ward suffering from the effects of burns – especially on her hands. The old lady and her husband lived in a small flat where a fire had started and they were both quite badly burned. When this happened the old man had been taken to a different hospital and had recovered sufficiently to come and see his wife. He was a small, bent old man, who walked with a kind of shuffle. He used to sit beside his wife and neither would utter a word. Sometimes the old lady asked her husband to get something out of her locker. In his tottering way he found what she wanted and they continued to sit in silence. Occasionally, the old man popped a sweet into her mouth, because she could not use her hands much.

One of the patients in the ward commented to Sister on the fact that the old couple hardly spoke to each other. Sister, with one of her rare humane touches, replied, 'They don't have to – they have been together for so long, they know what each is thinking without speaking.' I do not know whether the old couple had no family or whether they had outlived them, because nobody came to see them. This story has a rather more happy ending, as the old lady got well enough to go home. She was very low at one time and might easily have died through shock. The day came when the old man came to take his wife home. With the help of one of the nurses, he packed her belongings into a very ancient basket. We all wondered how they managed at home since they were both very feeble. With Nurse carrying the basket, the entire ward watched as they walked out together – again in complete silence.

My illness was now in its fourth year. Human nature, being what it is, still made it possible for me to indulge in wishful thinking. For example, how I might awake one morning and find myself better. With one swoop, how all problems would solve themselves and I would once more be reinstated as a useful member of society. This was to take place swiftly, painlessly and without top-level decisions about final operations. I think all this day-dreaming was good for me since it took me out of the hospital, so to speak.

I was smartly returned to reality by the words of the specialist who, on his next visit, said, 'There are no miracles – something else will have to be done.' Having said this he announced arrangements for another operation in two weeks' time. He was precise about the day, on a Friday, and the time 2 p.m. It was all terribly final and a great worry. During the next two weeks, the nights, always very long in hospital, became even longer. I seriously considered the prospect of death, which seemed to me a better alternative than failure. Going down under an anaesthetic seemed as good a way of dying as any for, as I have said elsewhere, it always felt a kind of death to me.

There had recently been a conversation in the ward about death. Death and laughter were strange bedfellows. One of the ward patients made everybody laugh when she pointed out that Sister managed to muster up a little respect for dead patients which she never found for living ones: from this it might be concluded that a corpse was no longer a patient. Occasionally the ward patients, finding nothing better to talk about, indulged in this type of gallows humour. Sister laid down her own code of behaviour. She did her duty and more for the patients but, like 'the Squire and all his relations', patients also had 'to keep to their proper stations'. Sister showed great deference to people in a greater position of authority than herself and towards the aristocracy. She was a staunch royalist and very proud of the fact that the matron of this hospital was invited to the Queen's garden party and ate strawberries and cream at Buckingham Palace.

Returning to the prospect of the next operation. It was terribly final. Until now I had somehow believed there was still a margin for error or failure, but the gap was now closing. If this coming operation was unsuccessful, I would be classed the same as Milly – that is, outside the pale so far as surgery or any other treatment was concerned. I read about those who faced troubles just as bad as mine or even worse, yet they rose nobly to the occasion and were not plagued by the thoughts that went on inside my head. Somehow, I was unable to measure up to those people.

I was rarely given medicine. Prior to the operation I was prescribed special medicine and was much intrigued by the name. It was called tincture of opium. Many novel and short-story villains were then depicted as silent, opium-eating men from the Far East, full of vice. The very word 'opium' conjured up a lurid, malevolent, sinister connotation. And I was now drinking it as an adjunct to healing – the word took on a new look.

The next two weeks seemed to pass very slowly. I was irritable during visiting times and not much help to my family, who were also feeling the strain. However, towards the end of this fortnight I started to feel better. I possessed a secret reserve of energy which could surface when needed, so that when the day of operation finally arrived, I felt better than I had anticipated.

On my way up to the theatre I was more than usually wide

awake. I caught a glimpse of the anaesthetist, whom I always regarded with great fear – as a kind of natural enemy. Gowned and masked in dead white, the general effect of which blasphemously reminded me of the Ku Klux Klan, he proved to be a very charming and sympathetic man, who really did his best to make the onrush of the ether feel less violent. He engaged me in conversation and when I asked him not to give me the anaesthetic too quickly, he earnestly agreed to do exactly as I wished, assuring me he would not even start until I told him to do so. I found his attitude helped to allay my fears, since it gave me a short time in which to adjust. However, in spite of his care and attention, the anaesthetic inflamed both my eyes and part of my face.

Sister told me it had been a long operation and I received similar reports from other people in the ward who told me, 'You were gone for ages.' It took me almost a week to recover from the first after-effects. I had no idea what had been done or what was likely to happen. All I did know was, for the first time I was left alone; that is, left alone in the sense that whatever had been done during the operation was being allowed to heal of its own accord. This was a great relief. With all the usual side effects of vomiting and pain, I simply hoped for the best.

When Sister appeared more communicative than usual about happenings concerning this last operation, it came as a surprise. Sister volunteered the information of her own free will. Not that it could be otherwise, for patients who had the audacity to ask questions about themselves received short, pithy replies such as, 'Mind your own business, it has nothing to do with you.' So that I listened with interest, when Sister told me that the doctor from the council hospital had been invited to attend, which he did. Also, that the specialist gave a short speech in the theatre, in which he disassociated himself entirely from all previous surgery, making it quite clear that I had arrived at this hospital in the present condition, adding that the reputation of the hospital was at stake. (It seemed the slight detail of my own future being at stake, was overlooked in this impassioned speech.) As the wound was surrounded by a large area which resembled a severe burn, it was impossible to incise it for surgery, so that the main incision had to be made well away from the inflamed region. The most interesting piece of news Sister gave me was that the trouble was entirely due to a breakdown of the surgery after the last major operation, performed by the doctor in the council hospital. Perhaps this was in the nature of an accident which might have happened to any surgeon, or there may have been other reasons. It is impossible for me to comment, other than say that I know the doctor there was as keen to be successful as the staff here.

There were no means of knowing any of this beforehand since, as I have already said, X-rays showed nothing. Therefore it in no way detracts from what the specialist did for me. So far as the operation was concerned, he did no more than any other competent surgeon might have done, but all honour must go to him because he did so when no one else would take the risk. The following incident will better help to illustrate this point. While I was in the council hospital, the ward doctor brought an outside surgeon to see me. Both doctors stood discussing my illness in medical terms which I did not understand, though I understood readily enough the reply given when the ward doctor suggested trying further surgery. The visiting surgeon said in no uncertain terms, 'I wouldn't touch it.' With the available knowledge of the history of this illness, it certainly seemed a risk. Yet this specialist undertook it on compassionate grounds and, in the face of considerable opposition by other doctors, he backed his own judgment.

There are times when medicine and nursing are so stimulating, exciting and rewarding, that the term 'sensational' is not an exaggeration. It is small wonder that many writers have drawn on this background for subject matter. I arrived here bedridden and in low spirits, with a condition regarded as pretty hopeless. Watching myself getting better, following the sudden and dramatic changes brought about by surgery, was as exciting as any thriller. After the first week the top dressing was changed, though the actual result of the operation was not revealed for almost two weeks after it had been performed. Everybody who was involved and a considerable number of members of the staff whom I did not know, came to see what the result looked like. The excitement was almost more than I could bear. The entire scene might have been part of a fascinating film, without any special actors – for people just to be themselves, was all that was needed.

During this period I had to keep a very tight rein on myself. For a short time I had been better before, though it did not last. I was haunted by this at first, unable to pretend it had not happened. My feelings divided between happiness and fear, I found it very hard to maintain an equilibrium.

As patients were then kept in bed after surgery much longer than at present, it was five weeks before I started to get up. I attempted to walk as best I could. Rehabilitation and aftercare were then unknown terms. It was taken as a matter of course that my legs did not carry me and my spine seemed too weak to support my body. No one thought there was anything special about the situation and the standard comment was, 'What can you expect, look how long you have been in bed!' Patients often look very different in bed and cause surprise when they are up and about. This applied to me for many expressed astonishment that I was not very tall; apparently lying in bed, I gave the impression of height which I did not possess.

Trying to walk was a great effort. At first, I had help from the nurses and later attempted to walk the distance from one bed to another by myself. I was spurred on by the feeling that once able to walk reasonably well, I could get out of hospital. It was not as easy as that. The large discrepancy between what I wished to do and what I was able to do, became more evident daily. Through not using my limbs I developed quite serious side effects. Some of the difficulties such as heavily swollen legs righted themselves after a short time, but another of those secondary conditions made life a burden for years afterwards. I do not know whether anything could have been done, for it is always a problem when secondary complaints are over-laid by a main illness. However, even the possibility of this was neither admitted nor discussed – all I needed was time. Again, it was a question of how things were viewed, rather than calculated neglect.

The transition from teens to twenty had changed me a great deal, for I had grown up in hospital. Therefore, it was not surprising that I possessed very little to wear, and what I did have did not fit me. Not that I was troubled about clothes at this stage, for I was much more concerned with trying to walk better. It was the gift of a dress for me which brought the question of clothes to the fore.

Among Sister's friends were a husband and wife; upper class and very well known in the area as voluntary social workers. They often came into the ward to have a word with Sister who behaved charmingly towards them, and the way Sister behaved was always a good index as to status and income group. The man, very tall, fair and distinguished looking, was afterwards knighted. There was something eccentric about his wife, which was reflected in the clothes she wore. She had a style all her own – totally unconnected with current or any other recognized form of fashion. Years later I was taken to visit the organization run by the lady and her husband. I was amazed to see numbers of young girls dressed in red jerseys and voluminous, bright red pantaloons. Much intrigued by those very strange costumes, I first thought they were taking part in a play. Later, it was carefully explained to me that the girls were wearing gym. costumes – especially designed by the lady herself.

One of the ward nurses told me an interesting story about the lady in question. She met with an accident serious enough for her to be admitted into hospital and insisted on coming into the general ward. There are various progressions of martyrdom and hers was one of not going into the private wing of the hospital. I suppose this kind of inverted snobbery was tied up with her social work. While in the ward she painted pictures which Nurse rather rudely described as 'frightful daubs'.

I must digress to say more about the above-mentioned nurse, whose name was Richards. She was fair, with a most elegant figure and altogether very feminine-looking; also clever, as she won prizes at the nursing examinations. With her dry and humorous way of telling a story, she told me that all the nurses of her year were instructed never to shout at patients in the private wing: as she hastened to point out, the logical conclusion was that it was quite in order to shout at patients in the public ward. And another memory of Nurse Richards. There was an aged, quite famous specialist at this hospital who maintained and campaigned for his pet theory, namely, that the colon was the main seat of infection in the body. He came into the ward unexpectedly one day and she gravely reported to the staff-nurse that 'bowels on the brain' was in the ward.

To return to Sister's friends. One morning the lady came to see Sister and they were both earnestly engaged in conversation – little did I know it concerned myself. It transpired later they were planning combined operations to make me a dress, as a gift – one in which I could go convalescent. This idea was rather a kindly thought. Sister told me they had bought some brown material for this dress as they thought it a good, serviceable colour. During the coming week, the material was duly delivered to the ward from one of the large stores.

Surrounded by an admiring audience comprising the nurses and other patients, Sister showed me the material. I hope that I said all the right things. The material was woollen, patterned and rather heavy. I gained the impression it was chosen for its durability and intended to last a long time. As I have already pointed out, the lady's own garments were rather strange and did not conform to any modern design, so that I was vaguely worried as to how the dress would look when finished. Neither did I know how far Sister's influence would go in relation to ordinary clothes since I had never seen her out of uniform and, after all, she was a product of the Nightingale era.

The lady and Sister must have been very industrious, for less than a week later the finished dress, packed in a large box with layers of tissue paper, was duly presented to me. I profusely thanked all concerned. An afterthought seemed to strike Sister for she suddenly said, 'Do try the dress on so that we can *all* see what it looks like.' I went back to my corner, carefully pulled all the curtains round my bed and started to get into the dress. (All hospital patients lived under conditions where 'modesty' was unknown. By virtue of their training, the medical staff hardly bothered about the niceties of patients being covered or out of range of full view. However, if a patient was dressing or undressing for reasons unconnected with medical matters, all bed curtains had to be drawn – by strict order.)

When I eventually managed to get into the dress, I could not believe it had been made especially for me. Very tight in the bodice, with yards of material in the skirt which made it very heavy. Although I could only see the front of the dress, the back felt inches longer – or was this intended as an uneven hemline? My natural shoulder line bore no relation whatsoever to the shoulders of the dress and the neckline pulled in conflicting directions. I emerged from behind the curtains to a stunned silence. This silence must have meant different things to different people for Sister thought I looked ravishing, though I was unable to share her enthusiasm. I was obliged to wear this dress when I went convalescent but never, ever, wore it again in public. If this sounds ungracious and ungrateful since everybody meant well, I can only take refuge in the fact that the dress had to be seen to be believed. Later, when I was home and felt low, I used to put on this dress and it never failed to make me laugh or raise a laugh from the family.

I was not in hospital much longer after this. Arrangements were in progress for me to go convalescent, though I still walked slowly and with difficulty.

There was no doubt that the specialist felt genuinely pleased when he came into the ward to see me for the last time. (I did actually see him just once more when I returned from convalescing – there was no further follow through.) He had a look at me and said laughingly, 'You know, any blooming thing might happen to that!' I received this gambit with mixed feelings. As usual, Sister spoke on behalf of the patient and told him I was having considerable muscular pain. The description was Sister's and not my own. In reply to her question as to why I could not walk any better, I said that it was the best I could do because of the pain. The specialist, continuing his conversation with Sister, suggested it might be a rheumatic condition and instructed the house surgeon to write up some medicine for me. (I think it was salicylic acid.) When the doctors had gone, Sister said it would be a good idea if I took the medicine with me to the convalescent home and then asked whether I could manage to go downstairs to the hospital dispensary, to have it made up. I was always pleased to go anywhere that made a change from the ward scenery. This happened on my last day in hospital when I had been formally discharged, so that the prescription was made out as from outpatients – which changed the rules.

The dispensary was in the hospital basement and seemed in the very bowels of the earth. First I tried walking down the stairs, but found this unnerving as I could not keep my balance.

Negotiating stairs was always difficult, even for people who had been in bed short periods. So I decided to use the old-fashioned lift, which was as big as a modern room and trundled noisily downwards at snail's pace. When I reached the dispensary I found it a large, dreary place, with unending rows of dark brown, wooden benches, the seats of which looked very shiny although the polish was worn away. I was alone in the dispensary, yet I could almost see endless numbers of people perpetually shifting along, in order to hand in prescriptions and have medicines made up. At the far end was a section partitioned off, made from dark brown wood, with glass top panels. The presciptions were handed in and the medicines collected through a small wooden hatch. I politely knocked as this hatch was closed. No one replied, so I knocked again, this time the hatch was flung open by a man I presumed to be the pharmacist. I handed him the prescription which he took without a word and banged the hatch shut again. I sat down on one of the empty wooden benches to wait; I was also glad of the rest, as I found doing quite ordinary things a great exertion. Some minutes later the hatch opened and a voice said, 'Four shillings to pay.' It seemed there was a charge made for all outpatients' medicines. I had to say that I did not have the money. The medicine was promptly taken back and the hatch shut down with a bang. I was left in the empty dispensary trying to work out what happened. All this took place without one word of conversation or explanation.

I returned to the ward by way of the lift, needless to say without the medicine. Sister was busy and did not notice my return, though she later asked me whether I had collected the medicine. I was obliged to tell her what had occurred. Sister was furious, for once not with me as a patient but with a member of the hospital staff. She checked on my answer again, 'Do you mean to tell me that he took back the medicine?' I assured her I did not get as far as having received it in the first instance. It was quite simple –

no money, no medicine. No doubt the pharmacist kept to the letter of the law which was, all outpatients had to make a payment for medicine.

By what method the money was allocated I never discovered, but the ward carried a money float of five pounds. Sister angrily took the required four shillings out of the ward fund, told the senior nurse she was going down to the dispensary and was gone for some time. Eventually she returned to the ward with the medicine, which she handed to me without speaking. With certain notable exceptions, Sister had scant respect for people – I wondered how she tackled the situation.

On the day I left hospital, the house surgeon had an enthusiastic pep talk with me. Among other things he said, 'Once you are convalescent you will soon pick up, be able to come home, find a job and start work.' The physical and mental repercussions of an illness lasting as long as mine were not mentioned, for the simple reason they were not admitted to exist.

This was in 1932. There was an all-high level of unemployment with conditions so bad that to be able to say one was working, was considered more important than health or anything else. It was the top priority. Young people leaving school at the age of fourteen were considered lost if they could not find a job before they were fifteen. Seven-year apprenticeships at low wages were a common form of cheap labour for those fortunate to be in work, with the prospect of learning a skill. In many cases young people left school without the hope of finding work – entire families were unemployed for years on end. The position of hospital housemen was commensurately just as bad. Grossly overworked and underpaid, with hardly any free time, their salaries were in the region of two pounds ten shillings a week, all found. It is fairly recently that young doctors have formed their own organization to better conditions. I mention those facts because the medical and allied professions lived in a closed society and seemed poorly informed about economic and social conditions. Thus, having turned twenty, hardly robust, without a skill, the house surgeon thought it should be quite a simple matter for me to find work – he foresaw no obstacles. He was a kind young man and I am sure that he meant well. When I pointed out I had been ill and out of circulation for the best part of five years, the house surgeon dismissed the problem completely and said arily, 'What's five years.'

Some hours later I left the hospital to go convalescent, having had a tremendous send-off with more good wishes than I could count. In the excitement I almost forgot the weird garment I was wearing, in the shape of the gift dress.

Going through my mind were all the events that happened during this illness. How at first, I could not believe I was ill enough to necessitate my having an operation – how for years I truly believed I would get better and later – the sudden realization that I was regarded as chronically and hopelessly ill – I remembered the first taste of freedom when I was better for a few short weeks – I thought about the amazing sequence of events, which culminated in that final consultation and the specialist deciding he would take a chance with me – how I was never forgotten by my family and, above all, the untiring efforts of my mother, in the face of every possible disadvantage.

Such were the thoughts that kaleidoscoped through my mind. Different people might call it different names, such as luck, chance, fate, or answers to prayers. With so many people to thank, I was conscious of an overwhelming feeling of good fortune – like someone who won on the millionth chance. At that stage I did not think about the future. I was only aware the greatest hurdle had been overcome and nothing that might happen afterwards could be as difficult.

Looking back on my life this summing-up still stands and I think of it as a victory.

8

I SPENT the next two months at a convalescent home which is now considered very close to London, but at that time was very much part of the countryside. It was a curious place, part comfortable and part with the dead hand of 'Institution' written all over it. There was a ward for bedridden patients, some of whom remained for long periods, though not indefinitely. The ground floor sitting-rooms were comfortably furnished with plenty of easy chairs and two couches. The upstairs dormitories were very large and, being insufficiently heated, always very cold. The beds were spaced out as in hospital, except that there were no dividing curtains or partition of any kind and underneath each bed was a large, oblong, wooden crate with slats all round, intended for the patient's belongings. The only other article of furniture in the dormitory was a small wooden chair beside each bed. As there were never quite enough to go round and at least two would always be missing, there were constant complaints from those who found their chairs missing. As for the best part of two weeks I was minus a chair, I became adept at doing what the others obviously did, namely, to seize the nearest chair from an unguarded bed and claim possession. Apparently this system worked quite fairly since it ensured everyone had a chair at least some of the time. There was a large, dreary dining hall, set with long trestle tables, and the food served therein reflected the atmosphere of the place. Although the concoctions served at meal times were different, the food came up in various shades of grey and always seemed to look the same. The meat for dinner was dark grey, as was the slice of sausage meat often served for supper, the potatoes a paler shade of grey and the vegetables cooked in such a way as to appear a greyish hue; the semolina, rice or bread and butter pudding always served as a sweet, were distinctly grey. The dining hall had two other memories for me. The first concerns an elaborate rota worked out consisting of a group of four patients whose job it was, every so often, to peel potatoes for the kitchen cook. In order to present themselves in the kitchen by ten in the morning, the names of the four patients were solemnly read out before breakfast started. I understand there were very few exemptions from this rota. The first time I was included in the group of four, as I entered the kitchen I noticed that the potatoes were on the floor, in a receptacle which resembled a medium-sized bath. With the other three I was handed a rather blunt knife and asked not to cut off too much potato peel, as this was wasteful. The other memory is that of grace before meals which we all repeated together so that the words 'For what we are about to receive may the Lord make us truly thankful' acquired a volume and power which I cannot easily forget, since there were well over a hundred people here. About a quarter of a mile down the road was the village where those able to walk and afford the cost, used to have tea or a meal every day. By far the nicest part of this entire place were the gardens. Even in bad weather the grounds looked attractive, as these were landscaped and carefully tended with a great profusion of trees, shrubs and flowers.

There were people here from almost every hospital in London, all women and ranging in age from fourteen onwards. The large number of young people reflected the pattern in hospitals at that time. Among the young were a considerable number encased in massive plaster casts for long periods who remained either in wicker spinal carriages which were full length or in wheel chairs; a few managed to walk slowly, notwithstanding the rigidity of the plaster casts. They must have felt weighted down and to add to their discomfort, the plaster might sometimes be left on too long and smell like decayed vegetation.

When this happened the patient would go back to the hospital for three or four days and then return to the convalescent home. All had bone diseases and not, as I first imagined, fractures. Although renewing plaster was not one of the things this convalescent home could do, there were very few places such as this, with a resident doctor and quite good medical facilities. I thought at the time how much more convenient it would have been for me here when the specialist at the hospital insisted on me going convalescent but no – I was sent to an entirely unsuitable place. Some of the patients here could have quite well afforded to take their convalescence where they wished, though what they might not readily have obtained was the medical or surgical treatment. Thus the patients were of a very varied background and kept very much to the groupings which tended to form as a result of social, economic and educational differences. However, all the things so far mentioned appeared of secondary importance. The really important part of this convalescent home was centred round the chapel and the most important person, the resident clergyman.

The clergyman was very short and always wore a cassock and an expression of permanent surprise. Although he did not speak a great deal he was much in evidence and would often appear quite unexpectedly – nobody having heard or seen him coming. He interviewed every patient, about whom he kept a record, and had one conversation with me on the day after my arrival. My conversation with the clergyman consisted of answers to several questions put in rapid succession. He asked me, 'Are you Church of England?' To which I replied, 'No.' He continued, 'Are you non-Conformist or Catholic?' To which I also replied, 'No.' I was just about to tell him I was Jewish when he said, 'Ah, you must be Greek Orthodox.' By this process of elimination, when my religious denomination had finally been established, the clergyman looked more surprised than ever and added I would be welcome at the chapel service any time I wished to attend. There the conversation ended. I inquired of some of the other people whether their conversation with the clergyman had been as short as mine. It appeared in most cases the interviews were even shorter, for if the answer to the first question ('Are you Church of England') was 'Yes', he simply said, 'I hope to see you at the services,' and no further word was uttered.

I went to the service on Sunday and was surprised at the large number of people present, some in beds, others in wheel chairs and wicker spinal carriages. Actually there was absolutely nothing to do on Sundays. The village, I was informed, was as good as dead for everything was shut and anyway it was made out of bounds for the day. Nothing was allowed on Sunday so that everyone came to the church service. Well, almost everyone. There were a group of five working-class women who never attended the service saying they never went to church anyway and had no intention of breaking their record. It was quite a good service – especially the communal hymn singing. The congregation definitely enlivened the clergyman and not the other way round. I have always considered the Sunday service performed an important function at the convalescent home, for it gave the religious section what they wanted and provided at least one Sunday activity for the rest of us.

Progress seemed very slow. The first two weeks I was told by the doctor not to get up until the afternoon. I struggled to improve my standard of walking by trying to do longer distances each day. After being up for a couple of hours and walking short distances I felt like crawling back into bed. Once up, this was not allowed. As in hospital, one could sit down but not lie down. The doctor here was young and very attractive and only the second woman doctor I had seen all the time I was in hospital. After I had been here a few days she said to me, 'I have received a special letter from the hospital telling me all about you and I gather you are rather wonderful.' 'I have been very fortunate,' was my reply to this unexpected description. I suppose it all depended on what the doctor meant by 'wonderful'. After all the excitement when I left hospital, I was now having a reaction and felt very depressed. The reason for this was two-fold. It was partly due to a feeling of worry as to what I was going to do when I went home and also to a vague uneasiness as to what was happening at home. I had no idea as to how long it would be before I could attempt working and, since I had neither skill nor a job, it seemed rather silly to worry in advance about a situation which was by no means clear. Yet I dwelt upon this aspect, wondering how I would shape up to a new life. I was frightened. The feeling of loneliness among a crowd was very acute here. Everyone had their own problems. Many were far worse off than myself without a hope of ever competing with the outside world, so I tried to console myself that it was something to have even reached my stage of worry.

As this convalescent home had a sick ward and some patients stayed for quite long periods, there was an organized system of visiting, which was unusual for these places at the time. Many of the people here had visitors regularly. I secretly hoped that someone from home would manage to come and see me for, although I had letters from home, nobody came to see me. At first I thought it might be due to the distance and expense involved and later started to feel vaguely worried that perhaps there was trouble at home about which I was not told. Knowing Mother, I found it hard to believe she would not have managed to come and visit me, at least once. I used to see the convalescent doctor every week and when at the end of seven weeks she suggested I could go home, I was very pleased. Firstly, I was very miserable at this place and secondly, I was unable to rid myself of the worried feeling that there was trouble at home. The doctor had given me a definite date for going so that when she sent for me two days later and said, 'We have decided to keep you here another week,' I was both surprised and frightened. I asked the doctor what difference another week would make and she said, 'Don't you want to spend one more week with us?' I hastened to add politely that it was not a question of me not wanting to stay as the fact the date of my leaving had already been fixed, so why was it being changed. The doctor then said, 'Well, we have received a letter from your mother asking us to keep you here just one week longer, because it is not convenient for you to arrive home on the date previously arranged.' I was unable to continue the conversation because the doctor had many others to see, though as I went out of the surgery, the worried feeling which had so far been vague, had now become positive. I was now sure something was wrong as I mulled over the words of the doctor. 'Not convenient for me to go home?' I could not believe it. 'Why?' The doctor obviously knew the truth but would not speak. So I stayed a further week during which time I received a letter from my young brother telling me that he would be coming down to see me home.

I could hardly sleep at night trying to work out what had happened at home and to whom. At first I decided Mother might have fallen ill and then thought it might be my father, whom I had not seen for months, was very much worse and perhaps could not be left. So the week crawled by, and at last came the day my brother would come. I had packed my few belongings hours ago and lay on one of the couches in the convalescent day room, to wait until he arrived. There was an affection between my brother and myself so that when I first saw him, I could tell he was ill at ease and worried. We were very pleased to see each other and I started the conversation by asking, 'How is everyone at home?' My brother's reply came rather slowly, 'Oh, all right, except for Dad.' There was a pause and I felt myself getting into a panic and afraid to inquire further. I pulled myself together and at last said, 'What's the matter with Dad?' Uneasily my brother replied, 'He's very ill and . . .' His voice trailed off. Suddenly I turned on him. 'Look, I'll have to know what's happened, so tell me the truth.' 'All right I will.' His words faltered as he said, 'Dad's been dead over a week.' I became silent trying to come to terms with the inevitable shock and finality of this last statement. Everything that had happened to me was driven from my mind and I was trying to anchor my thoughts to something tangible. My brother's next words probably did more to mitigate against the shock than anything else and I have never forgotten them. He said, 'Look, Belle, you know what Father's life was like and I saw him when he was dead – take my word when I tell you he looked more peaceful than he ever looked when he was alive,' I knew this was true.

All this conversation took place quietly whilst my brother and I were sitting on the couch where I had waited for him. There were several other people in the room though I do not think anyone heard what we said. As I said before, this convalescent home was very large with more than a hundred people, so I had already said goodbye to those whom I knew including the lady doctor. She assured me, as the doctor at the hospital had done, that all the physical difficulties would right themselves in due course and the memory of all that had happened would recede into the mist of time. The day was cloudy and grey though it was not cold. My brother had brought a warm scarf for me to wear. I put this round me as my brother took my case containing my belongings. We went out together to wait for the green country bus, which stopped right outside the grounds of the convalescent home, to take us to the station. I took a last look at the grounds, which were the only pleasant memory of this place – as usual, these looked delightful.

On the way home my brother told me how Father's death was unexpected. Although he was obviously very ill, he did manage to get up every day and for the time being it seemed that the pattern would be the same as other winters; that is, he would start improving as the weather became warmer. Mother had said he did not seem worse on his last night than he had been other times, so that when about eight in the morning he quietly died, it came as a shock. I said to my brother, 'Do you think Father knew that he was dying?' My brother replied, 'I'm certain he knew but, you know how he was – he never complained.'

When we arrived Mother was home by herself and she looked strained and ill. My home-coming was an anti-climax. In a curious way it was a non-event. Mother cheered up a little when she saw me and asked how I was. I remember sitting in the corner of the room feeling like a stranger who had arrived into a bereaved family by accident. Not that my father was unreal or remote to me, although I had not seen him for months. It was just that I had become estranged from my own family. Although the ties were never broken, somehow the pattern had changed and I felt I did not properly belong to the family group. Next day my aunt arrived. I have already mentioned she was Mother's younger sister and we were all very fond of her. My aunt spoke to me at great length and ended her conversation by addressing the rest of the family and saying, 'One thing about Morris (my father), he had the privilege and due of being able to die in his own bed, in his own home.' On this last point Mother agreed absolutely. I started to think about all the people I had seen die in hospital among strangers, sometimes quite alone although, of course, the one thing I had learned early during my illness, was that ultimately everyone dies alone, no matter how many other people are present. I had seen so many people die in hospital and my father had died at home where he belonged and among his own family. My aunt was right, though somehow I felt I also should have been home.

This feeling of estrangement from my own family was something I could not shake off. From a logical point of view it seemed almost ludicrous, after the years of struggle to get me home. In spite of the death of my father, we still seemed to be a family unit, yet I did not feel I belonged. If the feeling was unique, then so were the circumstances. At the time I neither described nor discussed this feeling with anyone else, partly because I was unable to easily put it into words and also because I thought others might disbelieve it. I was troubled for months by this sensation of being a stranger and it lessened only very gradually. Each morning I awoke with the idea I was in hospital and not in my home – it took me some time to readjust. By the afternoon I had once again integrated myself as a member of the family, yet the scene would repeat itself in exactly the same way next morning. This experience was frightening though I was powerless to prevent it. I was also somewhat irritated by the attitude of other people towards me, though I am certain they meant well. Roughly, they fell into two groups: the cheerful ones who said, 'Aren't you glad to be home – there is only one thing now and that is to look forward to the future, you have all your life in front of you, etc.,' and the others who commented, 'I suppose you became so accustomed to being in hospital that you can't believe you're home.' A long illness is always a traumatic experience and I went through many stages of readjustment. In fact I have only recently stopped having nightmares, when I would dream with such vividness that I was back in hospital with all the pain and misery, I literally woke up in a cold sweat to check on myself to see if I was holding together. It always took me a long time to compose myself after such dreams and I rarely went off to sleep again – somehow I felt safer awake.

The house in which we lived was about a hundred and fifty years old, with a deep cellar scullery and large rooms with very high ceilings, all in a hopeless state of disrepair. When I came home all this seemed very cramped to me, as I had become accustomed to living in vast hospital wards, so that the largest room seemed small by comparison. I could not settle down and all kinds of incidents long forgotten came back to me. Looking at the kitchen window I remembered how my brother and I had caused a lot of trouble in the following way. All the windows in the house were large with hinged window sills which opened like the lid of a long, narrow, oblong box. Inside was a huge wooden shutter which could be drawn up and fitted exactly into the window frame. Mother never used those shutters which she regarded with horror as she said they made her feel entombed. As children we used to play around with the shutter by lifting it part of the way up, and it went down all right, except on a particular day when my brother and I, having succeeded in getting the shutter to the top of the window, found it had jammed and we could not get it down again. Mother was most annoyed with us, as she could not get it down either. The kitchen light had to be on in broad daylight which was considered a wicked waste, while we waited for several hours for my father to return home; he, after a great deal of manipulation, managed to get the shutter down again with a terrific crash. I used to emerge from those fits of day-dreaming and think about the terrible gap in our family caused by the death of my father, and the great feeling of loss.

One of the first things I did when I came home was to compose a letter of thanks to the specialist. I use the word 'compose' advisedly, for I spent a great deal of time on this letter. It was a delicate situation. I wished to maintain the meticulous balance of not appearing sentimental, yet conveying the feeling of deep gratitude which I truly felt. I wrote several letters, none of which reached the required standard which I set myself. As I have already explained, the sister or nurse always spoke on behalf of the patient, so that direct communication between the patient and the specialist was reduced to monosyllables such as 'yes' or 'no'. The specialist himself never uttered one word other than was essential and Sister was very careful when talking to him, never to allow herself an opinion of any description. (This was in direct contradiction to almost everybody in or connected with the ward, where she was uncontested and laid down the law all the time.) It was small wonder that I had difficulty in striking the right note and balance. I disapproved of all the letters I had written though I could not go on writing for ever and had eventually to send one. I chose one of the letters with which I was by no means entirely satisfied and sent it direct to the great man himself. I did not expect any further mention of this letter. However, I was to hear later that it was noted with great satisfaction, since the specialist made particular mention of it to Sister, who afterwards passed on the information to me. Sister told me about the letter on the one occasion I went to the hospital to see the specialist not in the Outpatients' department, but in the ward.

There was no systematic follow-up when I came out of hospital. Once home, after two months' convalescence, I was treated in exactly the same way as other short-term patients in the surgical ward who were classed as cured and told to come to see the specialist once in the ward. This used to be the recognized procedure. Sister duly sent me a postcard telling me, or perhaps a better word would be 'commanding' me, to visit the ward on a Wednesday morning in order to see the specialist. He was hardly a man to register powerful emotion, yet I could plainly tell that he was very pleased with me. To have succeeded in closing a wound of such long standing, he had every reason to feel pleased. (It was after this interview that Sister referred to the letter which I had sent the specialist and she stressed how pleased he was with it.) During this visit it was noted that I walked with difficulty, though no attempt was made to investigate this further: it was merely noted in passing. There seemed to be a united front on the medical side that, given time and patience, all would right itself. This was wishful thinking since no one was very clear as to why I was unable to walk properly. As it transpired with time and patience – thirteen years to be exact – things did right themselves, more or less. However, at the time this advice was proffered no one really knew what was likely to happen. The violent pains in my back and legs continued unabated, so a few weeks after this last visit I wrote to Sister asking whether I might be allowed to see the doctor again, as I felt ill. Sister replied making another appointment for two weeks later, again in the ward. Three days before this appointment was due I received another postcard from Sister bearing the following message: 'I hope you are absolutely certain that you are *really ill*, so as not to waste the doctor's time because he is a very busy man.' Thus threatened, I started to worry as to whether I was ill enough not to be considered as having wasted the doctor's time. I felt unable to assess the position and in the end, gave the whole thing up. I never went back to that hospital. For a long time I did not seek help, hoping I might get better, until the situation became unmanageable and it was obvious that I had developed a secondary illness of some kind. This was actually the beginning of a protracted and serious illness as a result of being in bed for such long periods. Over the years there were several diagnoses of what this illness was likely to be and the doctors finally settled for a complaint called ankylosing spondylitis.

If I had visions of myself leading a normal, active and healthy life, such ideas were being gradually dispelled. I was naturally delighted to be home and thought at first after a sufficiently long rest, there would be no reason why I should not enjoy life. Of course, there were difficulties, for my only income was the seven shillings and sixpence which I received as a permanent disablement benefit. For most of the time I was in hospital I had received this same amount and was not accustomed to having more than two or three shillings over. Each week in hospital I used to pay for newspapers and sundry reading matter. Other incidental expenses were notepaper and stamps as a large number of ex-patients used to write to me and I carried on a surprisingly large volume of correspondence: I often wished people would have come to see me instead of writing. I consoled myself with the fact that my present problems bore no comparison to the misery and loss of freedom I endured whilst in hospital. There was the difficulty of trying to find work still ahead of me, but I would cross that hurdle when I came to it. Nevertheless I was plagued with violent pains, with my back as stiff as a poker and the perpetual difficulty in walking. In conversations with myself, I used to counsel patience and tell myself it was impossible to throw off the after-effects of such a long illness all at once.

Following a more than usual prolonged attack of violent pain, I decided to go and see a local doctor. He said, 'What's wrong with you?' I explained, 'I have great difficulty in walking and am having a great deal of pain.' The doctor continued, 'How long have you been unable to walk properly?' I told him something about myself and when he heard of this long illness, he actually laughed. 'Well now,' he said, 'you can't expect to be able to jump over the moon after all that – it may take you a year or longer to settle down.' So I paid him his fee of three shillings, apologized for having bothered him and went home.

This illness with which I came out of hospital was becoming progressively worse although I continued as best I could for another few months. I then decided to go to a hospital which knew nothing about me and would give no details of previous illness unless directly asked to do so. The hospital I chose was an orthopaedic one and here the approach was better, especially when it was discovered I ran a temperature. I was very slow at dressing and undressing as the movements of my arms were also restricted, so that I found it difficult to perform the most ordinary actions, such as getting into shoes and stockings and combing my hair. The Outpatients' nurse said briskly, 'Hurry, my dear, you are keeping the doctor waiting.' The doctor went over me very thoroughly and, gazing at the scarring said, 'Now that must have been a battlefield.' How true, I thought, but said nothing. The doctor was not so easily put off as he continued, 'Now tell me a little more about this.' Condensing a five-year medical history into one sentence I said vaguely, 'Well, it started off as acute appendicitis and did not go according to plan.' 'What went wrong with the plan?' I was truthfully able to reply, 'I don't know.' The doctor then asked me which hospital I was in last and told me to come again the following week, as he wished to get some more information about me. Facilities in this hospital were primitive to say the least, so that the nurse once again implored me to get dressed quickly as others were waiting. (Years later, when I had a regular job, the girls at work used to help me re-do my hair and tidy up generally when I arrived in the morning.) The consultation between the doctor and myself took place in a large room with many other people waiting, and the various cross-conversations both between the nurse and the patients and the doctor and patient, sounded like a meeting in a public square.

The following week I went back to see the doctor. He read the report about me and not surprisingly looked a trifle vague. My hospital notes were very long and probably detailed, though they were never co-ordinated, with the result that if information was required by another doctor, it gave a not too accurate account of the different hospitals I had been in, complete with the number of operations and ended with the words, 'Now apparently quite better and able to work.' At the time this report was received – I read it myself as it was pinned to the top of my outpatient's card – the hospital knew nothing about me. Having left, there was no follow-up and they had no idea as to whether I was working or what I was doing. The orthopaedic doctor suggested I have X-rays taken to see whether this might show why I had difficulty in walking. For the plates to be taken and the report to come through took two weeks. When I returned to the hospital the doctor studied the X-ray plates and read the radiologist's report. Finally he told me I had arthritis in both hips and unfortunately there was little he could do about it. I remember asking the doctor, 'Won't I ever be able to walk better than this?' His reply was, 'I'm afraid not.' So ended the consultation. The doctor was very frank though the net result seemed to be that little was known and nothing was learned about the after-effects of so long an illness. However, I must confess I was not without sympathy for the doctors. To have to unravel a five-year history of illness where cause and effect were so inextricably interwoven, made it difficult to reduce this maze of information to manageable proportions. It was also a question of being interested enough. I know from experience that most doctors hate to be confronted with cases of this kind. They have no direct knowledge of the original illness and have to obtain the information from reports and what the patients happen to know about themselves; all this is very time-consuming and open to misinterpretation.

A great deal has been said and written about will-power in relation to illness. Like a lot of generalizations I suppose it is true in part, depending on the circumstances. When we were in the council hospital Milly and I used to sometimes discuss this aspect though when we tried to define will-power, we got into deep water. It seemed to mean so many different things, including determination, purpose, resolve, intention and control, etc. Well, we both had many of these attributes in good measure, most especially Milly, who had enough drive, determination and sense of purpose for several people, yet no degree of will-power could

6*

have made it possible for either Milly or myself to have overcome the original illness. However, I can truthfully say that I overcame the serious after-effects myself, for I had the greatest difficulty in getting doctors to believe this took the form of a specific illness. As I have tried to make clear, it was accepted as inevitable – rather like original sin. At a later stage this attitude modified somewhat and I had various forms of treatment, most of which made me worse. This was not surprising since there was a great deal of doubt and difference of opinion as to the nature of the complaint. I had to withstand not only the complaint, but also the cures. All this took a long time and I now walk normally. If the reader asks, 'What did I do?' The answer is 'Nothing'. I arrived at the stage where I knew there was only myself to rely on and if I was able to hold on long enough to withstand the intense pain – I would get better. This proved to be true though I do not know whether my attitude could pass as will-power.

9

THE changing world I encountered when I came out of hospital showed itself in all kinds of ways. There had been serious unemployment for years, though it was now at an all-high level, with grave repercussions on large sections of the population. Yet all manner of other changes were also taking place. The old clanking trams were being gradually replaced by buses. Radio sets had developed into sophisticated knob-twiddling designs. There were still many homes without radio, including my own; we did not aspire to this luxury until 1938. Hiking was a popular and inexpensive pastime – people walked for miles as a means of enjoyment. In this connection I recall Sister having a late summer holiday the last few months I was in hospital. When she came back on duty one of the doctors asked, 'Did you enjoy your holiday, Sister?' 'Very much,' said Sister enthusiastically. 'We walked a long distance every day and one day we covered twenty-five miles.' Sister was a seasoned walker for she had plenty of training in her daily duties. Strangely enough, I did not consider that distance very remarkable at the time. I was so accustomed to seeing the nursing staff walk back and forth across the ward, that twenty-five miles did not seem to me so way out.

The cinema was probably the most popular form of entertainment for the majority of the people. Large numbers of new cinemas were opening, bigger and better than their predecessors. A new cinema opened near to where I lived. It was extensively advertised for months beforehand and described with such adjectives as 'stupendous', 'sensational' and 'super de luxe'. It really looked lavish when it was finally opened with great pomp and ceremony. Standing outside the cinema was an enormous commissionaire. His brown and beige uniform was decorated with gold braid and gold buttons and, tucked into epaulettes on his left shoulder, was a pair of snow-white gloves: he would not have disgraced an Admiral of the Fleet. (I still pass this cinema which is now, alas, a disused warehouse, without even a glimpse of the glory that was.) While I was in hospital I read about the wondrous invention of talking pictures. These started showing in America in 1927. By the time they arrived in London I had already become ill, so that, when I came home from convalescence, I longed to get well enough to see a talking film. When I eventually accomplished this, I remember being so amazed at the technical changes involved, I hardly followed the story and to the present day cannot recall the name of the film. I know that I did not enjoy it, so great was the impact of change.

My greatest worry was how I was going to obtain work and, if I was lucky to get any kind of work, whether I would be able to do it. The permanent stiffness and perpetual pain went on round the clock, often reaching a point where, try as I might, I could not get out of bed. I varied not merely from day to day, but almost from hour to hour. Sometimes I would walk with rather less difficulty; other times my legs and back were so completely locked as to give an impression that I was carved out of one rigid piece, minus any joints that could bend. No one at home asked me how I was, since if I felt better in the slightest it became obvious, for I would go out for a walk or help Mother in the house. The same attitude towards pain obtained as it did in hospital. From time to time I did see various doctors and no one ever thought of asking how I coped with the pain or giving me anything for it. My morale was not as low as one might have expected, for I always consoled myself with the thought – I might have still been in hospital – after all, Milly was still there. I had been home about four months and decided to make some tentative inquiries in connection with trying to find work. I had to start somewhere and the interview I intend to describe, came about through a chance remark.

I was advised to try and obtain an audience with a lady who was an Honourable and who shall be nameless. I was told that she interested herself in people with personal problems and might be able to help. After further inquiries and correspondence I managed to get an appointment. This appointment was for the early afternoon when I duly presented myself at the arranged time. To see her I had travelled a considerable distance and climbed several flights of stairs, which I always found difficult. Somewhat breathless as a result, I remember sitting down on a highly polished mahogany seat in the corridor to regain my composure and think about what I was going to say to the lady. As I sat and meditated, a young woman came through one of the various doors and asked what I wanted. I told her that I had an appointment to speak with the Honourable lady and showed her the letter of confirmation, whereon she disappeared taking the letter with her. The young woman returned and beckoned me into another room which was an outer office, from which a door opened on to an inner office, where the Honourable lady sat. I waited another few minutes and was finally received into her presence.

The Honourable was a thin, almost gaunt-looking, woman who seemed to me quite old. I think she was actually considerably younger than she looked, though her clothes were so dowdy as to make her appear almost frumpish. I recall she wore a dark grey, ankle-length coat, brown flat-heeled shoes and brown lisle stockings. Her hair, streaked with grey, was combed down on either side of her face and drawn backwards into a bun. I was not at all clear as to what the Honourable lady precisely did, but thought she was probably a social worker, similar to the friends of Sister who helped make me the gift of the strange dress.

If I had been thinking hard about what to say it was a waste of time, for I was merely required to answer questions. The conversation which ensued went like this:

The Honourable: Have I seen you before?
Myself: Never before, Madam.
The Honourable: What exactly is it you want?
Myself: Any kind of help to find a job.
The Honourable: This is very difficult – you must surely be aware of the extensive unemployment.

Having always prided myself on my social consciousness and economic awareness, I was somewhat nettled by this last remark. However, the conversation continued.

Myself: Yes, I know about unemployment, but I am in special difficulty as I have not worked for years because of illness. I was in hospital nearly five years.

The Honourable: Five years! This is surely a long story and I have really little time.

There was a pause.

The Honourable, continuing: I take it then you have no skills of any kind?

Myself: No, but I'm sure I could learn.

At this point in the conversation there was an even longer pause. It seemed that the Honourable was considering the situation and went off into a trance-like silence. I just waited.

Presently the Honourable spoke and asked,

'Are you fond of children?'

This was a totally unexpected question.

Myself, somewhat vaguely: Well, I don't dislike them.

The Honourable: You do not sound very enthusiastic. I think that looking after children will be a splendid idea; I could place you in that capacity almost immediately, as I know someone with three young children who is in need of help. Of course, you would have to supply very good references.

Myself: I have no references from previous jobs.

The Honourable: Oh, I understand that – just references about character and disposition from people who know you such as a minister, your doctor or schoolteacher – anybody of some standing who has known you a long time.

There was another silence, after which the Honourable became even more animated and continued: 'This type of work could solve a lot of problems. First of all you could live-in, which means your mother will not have to worry about feeding you. Secondly, you will have plenty of fresh air, as the children must be taken out every day. Of course, all this depends on your references being first class and you making a favourable impression.'

All the time this conversation was going on, I felt my hackles rising. This woman seemed to have no comprehension of the true circumstances. Was it possible that she failed to grasp the fact that I had been away from home for nearly a quarter of my life? I had taken it for granted she would understand that my being home was something of a miracle. She assumed that going to live in a strange home and looking after three children would be a simple matter – that it was merely a question as to whether I could produce suitable references! This was leading nowhere. It was obvious she did not begin to understand what my problems were really like. I was quite unequal to the situation and woefully unable to make the situation plainer. Suddenly, I found all this so overwhelming, that I grasped the table to help me stand up as quickly as possible, said 'Good afternoon', walked through into the outer office and back down the stairs, the way I had come. The Honourable stared after me; she was genuinely amazed I had behaved in this way.

On looking back on this disastrous interview, I know that had I been older and a little more experienced I should never have run away. The onus was on me to have tried to break down the problem so that she might have understood. In the most favourable circumstances this was no easy task since we were separated by age, by class and by outlook. I had come in the first place to ask for help but had been unable to establish terms of reference. Although we both spoke the same language, we were unable to communicate.

When I arrived home Mother asked, 'And how did you get on?' Referring to the Honourable she said, 'I have heard she is a very nice person.' I replied rather shortly, 'She was quite nice but it did not lead anywhere.' My mother did not like 'do-gooders' and might have given me moral support had she known the details. I could not really justify my behaviour which was due to a lot of pent-up feeling inside me, so that I was unable to openly admit the failure. I felt that I had gone wrong somewhere and made a complete hash of the interview, so I did not want to elaborate. This was my first and last experience of asking for this kind of help. The whole episode was far less disastrous than I imagined, for it probably never could have led anywhere. Nevertheless, it did one very important thing for me. From then on, I knew that within the limits of what was possible, I would have to help myself and that there was no one else to rely on. Although this decision sounds simple, it really gave me a clear sense of direction.

My main pastime was reading. I rejoined the public library which had the disadvantage of being a long way from where I lived. It was quite an effort for me to walk there and I could only do this on the days I felt better. I used to do this walk by easy stages and have a long rest in the reference library when I finally arrived. This library had a huge room which displayed every national newspaper plus local papers. Most of the time I spent looking at the papers both for the news and also in the forlorn hope that I might be fortunate enough to get on to some work through one of the advertisements. This never materialized, since highly skilled workers and graduates were out of work in large numbers. I usually ended those sessions at the library by taking out two books to read at home.

As a result of an advertisement in the local press I did go after one job which was nearby. The advertisement in question was so vaguely worded it was impossible to elucidate what this firm really wanted – if they wanted anybody at all. When I arrived I found thirty or more other girls there, also in the hope of getting this job – whatever it was. Even the firm's name was vague for they styled themselves 'General Dealers'. The firm's manager interviewed everyone as I do not think he had anything else to do. It was impossible to glean any information about what they wanted because the girls who had already been interviewed must have used another way out, so we did not see them again. As there was nowhere to sit, I stood around waiting for over an hour. I decided the whole thing looked doubtful – perhaps a better word might be 'phoney' – and was on the verge of going home as I was so tired, when it became my turn to go in and be interviewed. The man who did the interviewing was young and very sure of himself; he started off by firing a whole series of questions. Did I understand anything about patterns? Was I adaptable enough to do other things (unspecified) if the occasion arose? What experience of any kind did I have? And finally, information about every other job I had worked in. By his side he had a large notebook filled with names and addresses and other entries which, no doubt, he thought relevant. I hardly need add that I did not stand an earthly chance. However, my name and address was duly entered in the large notebook and he ended the interview with the time-honoured words, 'I have many more people to see and will let you know.'

There used to be a great deal of advertising of this type. One wondered why those firms spent the money on advertising and what they really wanted.

Trying to obtain some kind of work was still my greatest worry. I had been home from convalescence for months and now realized the difficulty I had in walking was not going to right itself quickly, if at all. Our family, including my father, had been connected with the fur trade and it was in that industry I had started work when I became ill. It seemed logical at the time because I knew something of the trade generally and remembered fragments of what I had previously learned during the short time I worked. So it was, at the time of mass unemployment I was confronted not merely with trying to find a job, but having to learn a skill when I was past twenty.

The fur industry is seasonable and at its busiest during the summer months, so it was then that I went job hunting. I managed to find a job after a few weeks – a very bad one. The conditions of work were deplorable. The firm consisted of one room about the size of a large room in a private house, situated at the top of three flights of rickety, wooden stairs. It was in the vicinity of Goswell Road in the City, part of an area which was afterwards destroyed by bombing during the second world war. One corner of the workroom was partitioned off to serve as an office for the employer. This one room had three doors: one had the words 'Employees Only' painted on it in large, black letters; the second bore the imposing inscription, 'Office. Strictly Private. Please Ring Bell'; and the third door was on the inside, included in the partition which separated the office from the workroom. On the same floor facing the workroom were two dirty lavatories and a small, yellow, cold water sink, which seemed to be used by everyone else in the building as well as the fur workers. Inside the workroom there were two woodern benches fixed against the wall, successfully cutting off half the window space. The room also contained three fur machines, one flat machine and a pair of trestles, which supported a wooden board large enough to hold an entire fur coat, laid out flat. In one corner of the room stood a makeshift kind of table with a shelf near the bottom, at which sat several girls doing hand sewing. Close to this large table was a smaller one, on which stood several cracked teacups and a tin box, probably containing tea. On the floor at the side of this table stood a gas ring in a highly dangerous position. There were two men who stood against the bench cutting the furs, one man who nailed the coats on to the large board, and two undersized apprentice boys, who seemed at the beck and call of everyone; the rest of the staff were young women. The workroom was very crowded and very dirty, with an atmosphere like a furnace. The reason for this intense heat was the large coal fire burning on this summer morning, for the purpose of drying the fur coats, since these had to be stretched and tacked down while wet. Neither was it possible to open the windows very wide because the benches were in the way, so that each time the top of the windows were opened or closed, someone pretty agile had to jump up on the bench to do this. None of the girls who sat to do their work had other than a wooden stool without a back to sit on. When Robert Owen the reformer set up his factory in New Lanark at the turn of the eighteenth century he probably had superior working conditions to this place where I spent my first half day working in 1932. And this was by no means an isolated case, for there were large numbers of such workrooms in and around the city.

In my interview with the employer before I started this job, I pretended to know much more than was actually the case, knowing something of the trade terms. I did most of the talking and became so passionate and eloquent that I really began to believe what I said myself. The employer listened for a while and then said very shortly, 'Start on Monday morning' and he disappeared from view. This happened mid-week, so I spent several sleepless nights wondering how this job would work out. The answer is that it did not work out and I lasted only half a day. 'As you don't know anything about the work you're not expecting any pay, are you?' Those were the employer's last words and he did not expect an answer. However, even in that half day by watching the other girls, I managed to pick up one or two points which helped me in my next job, where I lasted one and a half days.

Some weeks later I got a third job, where I decided to try different tactics. I decided to take a chance, tell the employer something about myself and make a proposal to him: namely, that I was willing to work for nothing for a period, in return for learning something of the trade. The effect on the employer was quite different to what I had naïvely anticipated. He became highly suspicious of my motives and absolutely refused to enter into such an arrangement.

To say that I was tired when I arrived home after my first attempts at working, in no way gives a true indication of how I felt. I was prostrated. Stiff from unaccustomed sitting for hours at a time, it used to take me at least twice the normal time to reach home for I had to do this very slowly, step by step, holding on to the nearest wall to maintain my balance. I travelled to and from work by tram, which was usually packed to suffocation and mostly I had to stand all the way. This was actually better for me than sitting. One day, as a result of sitting in the tram, I could not get up when it came to the stop where I lived. I made several attempts, much to the curiosity of the other passengers, but was unable to get on to my feet, so, I continued travelling in the tram, The conductor, who was a lively cockney, said to me, 'What's the matter, luv – don't you want to go 'ome?' I intimated there was nothing I wanted more than to be able to go home – I could not get up. The conductor continued, 'Got a touch of the screws? Blimey,' he went on, 'at your age – what you going to be like when you get old?' He had a point. To continue this story to the bitter end, the tram terminus was at East India Dock road – miles from where I lived. I went right to the end of the journey, with the banter of the conductor going on all the time. ''Ave to charge you extra fare', he kept telling me. The seats on the trams were wooden and used to be reversible by sliding backwards. I came back on the same tram and eventually, with the help of the conductor, for the trams used to pull up almost in the middle of the road, I managed to get on to the pavement and somehow staggered home. My family was worried and wanted to know where I had been. 'To East India Dock,' I reported gravely. When I gave the details of the story to my family, we all laughed – it seemed to be the best way to take it.

Alongside all the difficulties I can also recall much kindness. I had a friend in the fur trade who helped me a great deal by answering my many questions. This type of theory linked with the practical side and helped to make things easier. Many years later when I started teaching others the trade, their difficulties were always very clear to me because I so vividly remembered my own. In those days there was little or no real tuition connected with work process. Highly skilled workers were never encouraged to pass on their skills to others. They were, in fact, afraid to do so, for the simple reason that they had no protection for their own jobs. One of the most sincere and really good people I met during this troublesome part of my life was Eva. I had been working on and off for a few months, never lasting more than days in each job, when I came across Eva in one of the larger firms where I had just started. She had been with the firm for many years. Very plump and very fair, she had a calm manner which nothing could disturb – she was unflappable. I had become very wary as to how much I told anyone about myself, since I had learned enough to know that the first prerequisite of any wage earner is to maintain good health. Workers not in possession of this asset are considered a bad risk by employers. Eva was very observant and noticed I was having difficulties. She could have made trouble for me, as the employer set great store by her judgment when assessing new workers. Without asking me questions, she had me moved next to her and not only helped me learn the job but quite often urged me to have a rest, while she did the work I was supposed to be doing. How often one hears the phrase 'It made me lose faith in human nature.' Eva was the finest antidote for this frame of mind.

What made it hard for me to keep up morale, was the dreary cycle of working a long day and having to spend the rest of the time in bed. Hours of work were generally from 8.30 a.m. until 6.30 p.m. with half day on Saturday. I used to get home too tired to eat and the first thing I did was to get into bed. Most week-ends I also spent in bed for it was impossible for me to keep going otherwise. I had no recreation. This went on for years. I could not make definite long term arrangements of any description, for I never knew whether I would be able to keep them. If it so happened I had a bad day arrangements meant nothing at all and would go by the board. My life was governed by the way I walked and how severe the pain.

When I first came out of hospital I was certainly prepared to give myself time to settle down. As time went by and I did not make the headway I expected, my first feeling was one of frustration. It made me furious to think that I had actually managed to reach the stage where I had my freedom and was liberated from the everlasting dressings and surgery, yet in a way I felt cheated. Later, it was not so much that my situation improved, as the fact I became more accustomed to this curious, uncertain mode of living and was better able to face it. Most people who knew about me were amazed I succeeded in finding the various jobs and that I was working at all. When I stopped to consider it I was surprised at myself. The times I did think about myself in this way was when I heard from Milly, who was still in the council hospital, in the ground floor ward where I had left her. During the four months I was home and not working, I used to go and see her on the days I felt better and able to do the journey. Milly was obviously very pleased to see me and used to say that she wished I could come more often. We talked 'shop' a great deal and she would tell me what was going on in the hospital. As usual, she was very up to date. She still made pincushions and several finished ones were always on her bedtable ready for sale. One day I asked her how she was faring and if there was any sign of change in herself. 'I'm as you left me – there's no change.' Her answer was short, I got the message and did not pursue the subject. I used to speak to those nurses whom I happened to know and noted some had become staff nurses and others sisters. The same sister was still on the ward and she urged me to forget the customary visiting times and see Milly whenever I was able to do so. During one of those visits I tried to explain to Sister the kind of trouble I was having in walking and began the conversation apologetically with, 'All things considered I hesitate to complain, but . . .' Sister listened carefully and said, 'Anything could happen after such a long illness.' She then added another interesting observation I had not heard anyone else mention. 'This wound was closed quickly by surgery – it was there one day and not the next – so that the re-direction of the bowel and the accompanying septic condition healed suddenly, which may have caused other repercussions.' There were other incidents when I went to see Milly. For example, I always found it an uncanny experience to be able to walk through the hospital gates, across the stone paved quadrangle to the ward, for it was in this area I used to stare through the ward window, making believe it was me outside and not some stranger. One afternoon on my way to visit Milly, I walked through the gates of the hospital thinking about something totally different. The bright red jumper and navy blue skirt which I was wearing felt definitely tight and uncomfortable. My sister had lent me these clothes and I managed to get into them although she was somewhat thinner than me, but somehow I felt sure it gave the tell-tale impression the garments did not belong to me. Engrossed in such mundane thoughts I suddenly came face to face with Dr Wilson, the hospital medical superintendent – the very doctor who had said of Milly and myself, 'those two girls ought to be in the "House", they occupy two beds to no purpose.' At that really dramatic meeting we both stood still and neither of us spoke. Without one word of recognition, looking at me very intently for Dr Wilson knew me well though it was about thirteen months since I had left the council hospital, the silence was long enough for the entire scene to re-enact itself about going into the workhouse and the dreadful thought of perhaps being lost forever. Having recovered sufficiently from being taken entirely off-guard, I continued to walk on towards the ward. Dr Wilson, never for a moment taking his eyes off me, watched me until I was right out of sight. When I reached the ward I sat down outside to consider the incident about which I had very mixed feelings and wondered why I never registered complete triumph. I thought it was because I had been better for a few weeks while I was in this council hospital and it had left me uncertain and cautious. As the nurse came over to tell me it was all right to go in and see Milly, I wondered what she would say when I told her of this strange meeting. When I told her she listened to this story without words with much interest and said, 'I'm jolly glad that happened – when he saw you he saw with his own eyes what was possible, which all helps to shake his cocksure attitude.' Neither of us had forgiven him for the workhouse incident. Milly laughed as she added, 'You know, I think Dr Wilson is foresworn never to speak to any patient, past or present.' Soon after this I started work and was too tired to make the journey to and from the hospital to see Milly, so we corresponded. I recall one letter in particular she sent me at the time, in reply to one I had written telling her that I had started work. Milly wrote, 'I read the one sentence again and again – you have really been able to start work! Isn't it wonderful and goes to prove almost anything is possible.' I did not elaborate on the difficulties I was having since everything is relative and she would have gladly undertaken all such difficulties in return for her freedom. Each time I heard from Milly it had a sobering effect on me for I thought, 'There but for the Grace of God, go I.'

Although the problems of the stifled and inhibiting atmosphere of life in hospital were mostly concerned with living or dying, and the problems of the world outside seemed eclipsed, yet they might be concerned with the same thing. When I started to lead a relatively normal life, the terrifying problem of unemployment overshadowed all else. And the word 'terrifying' is not too strong a term for mass unemployment, for this had a stranglehold on the nation when I first became ill and continued to a greater or lesser degree five years later when I began to look for a job. It was reflected in every aspect of the way the majority of people lived, even in the manner they conversed. The leading question of all conversations was 'Are you working?' If the answer was 'No', the usual gloomy conclusions were drawn: if the answer happened to be 'Yes', the implication was there was nothing whatsoever to worry about, since all other things were relegated to second place. This attitude certainly applied to me. I desperately tried to ignore all physical difficulties and concentrate on work. At least, the attitude applied in theory, for in practice I was no better able to walk than in the first weeks I was discharged from hospital. My mother urged me to try and get further medical advice, 'Before the illness becomes chronic,' she said. So I tried again and went to one of the large voluntary hospitals.

In order to attend this hospital I had to have time off work. This created a difficulty for, in spite of the fact that nobody in this firm was paid for time lost, it was difficult to obtain permission to have unpaid time off. I had to give a detailed explanation as to where I was going and why I needed time off. For want of a more accurate diagnosis I shortly described myself as having rheumatism. It so happened that the wife of one of the directors suffered badly from arthritis, so that if I did not receive any pay I received a certain amount of sympathy from him. Even this was useful. I started on a long, drawn-out course of treatment which meant going to the hospital three times a week. This treatment made me worse though the doctor insisted that if I persevered, things would improve. In all fairness no one at the firm complained about my having time off and the foreman was especially understanding. I started to worry. I was certainly not indispensable at work and, coupled with the loss of pay, after four weeks I told the doctor I would be unable to come any more. He was very sympathetic and said he would transfer me to a hospital with an evening clinic, of which there were several at that time. I am sure this was by accident and not design but the place to which he transfered me was a private clinic. When the secretary of the clinic told me the scale of charges I turned to go, since it was out of the question. It was a delicate situation. Perhaps not so much because I was unable to afford the clinic charges, as the fact that out of courtesy a doctor, having written a letter on behalf of a patient, usually needed a reply and it rather put the secretary in a position of having to point out to the doctor this was the wrong kind of clinic to have recommended. Or, it may have been a spontaneous gesture on the part of the secretary for, as I turned to go, she said, 'Don't go, since you are here perhaps the doctor will see you.' She asked me to accompany her and told me where to sit and wait. I waited for hours. Every one else came and went and I just sat and waited. Finally, there were so few people about I could see the clinic was on the verge of closing. I was considering whether to go back and speak to the secretary if she was still in the clinic, or just go home, when a doctor came walking down the corridor with a haughty-looking sister at his side. The doctor then addressed the sister and asked, 'Do you know why that girl is waiting?' He was obviously referring to me. The sister, after giving me a somewhat disdainful look, replied, 'Oh her, she came here with a letter from another hospital and it seems she can't even pay.' The inclusion of one short, rather insipid word, coloured the entire sentence. Had the Sister said, 'She can't pay,' it would have simply been a statement of fact. But it was the word 'even' – 'She can't even pay,' that succeeded in reducing me to the level of human beings totally outside the pale so far as Sister was concerned.

The doctor then did something which Sister did not anticipate. He said, 'I'll see her.' He told me to go along with him and actually returned to his consulting room, where he spent the best part of an hour questioning me and trying to get some kind of lead as to the reason I could not walk properly. He did not take the attitude that, having been in bed for years, it could not be helped. The doctor told me to come and see him again three days later and added, 'Don't worry about the money side.' Sister did not say anything, though I could tell she was surprised by the turn of events.

Three days later I returned to the clinic where I had an X-ray taken and made one subsequent visit. The doctor made one very important deduction, namely that the source of the trouble was not in my legs but in my spine. He transferred me to yet another privately run clinic with the words, 'The fact that I am sending you elsewhere has nothing to do with payment – it is because we do not have the apparatus to treat you here.' The doctor behaved very humanely towards me for this clinic was, after all, a private one and in no way bound by the system on which hospitals were run. I attended the second clinic for a long time, having the same difficulties in walking and moving as I had had all along. The specialist there had enormous confidence in his treatment (I think it was the result of his own researches) and made it the sole reason I continued living at all, for I quote him, 'If it were not for this treatment you would be kicking up daises.' If that doleful metaphor between daises and death was supposed to ram home to me the grim realities, I have to admit that it misfired. So far as I was concerned I still walked with difficulty and was unable to perform the most ordinary duties such as pulling on my stockings, lacing my shoes or doing my hair. I did not mention any of these details at the time because the specialist was really a very kindly man and I might have sounded grudging or ungrateful. This was not the first time I experienced these curiously unequal word contests in which the doctor became wildly enthusiastic and the patient remained thoroughly miserable.

This stubborn illness with which I came out of hospital continued for thirteen years. During those years I was back in hospital several times; it seemed that nothing could improve it. There was a stage when I seriously doubted my chances of ever getting well again, yet at the height of this depressive period and when I least expected it, the pain started to abate and I slowly but surely began to get better. I think this was a good example of the phrase sometimes used by doctors – especially when the patient does not respond to known treatments – namely, 'time is the greatest healer'.

When I finally became a skilled worker I gained confidence and obtained a job with very good working conditions and where I remained for the next thirty-five years, the rest of my working life. As a mink machinist I learned the trade in a very hard school, sometimes, in the early days, working under the most appalling conditions. If I wished to earn the top rate of pay I had to maintain the maximum output. There were no allowances made and no quarter given. The advantage this early period offered was that I handled every known fur, which gave me a thorough all-round knowledge of the trade. The work was hard and tedious with most of the girls complaining of feeling tired, though I used to start work tired and towards the afternoon I had the greatest difficulty in keeping going at all. Over the years there have been changes both in conditions of work and the availability of jobs. As in many other industries pressure through trade union representation on the Wages Council succeeded in gaining, among other things, pay for statutory holidays and three weeks annual holiday with pay. I have been one of the workers' representatives on the workers' side of the Fur Wages Council for many years and, looking back recall the passionate arguments on the employers side on behalf of the very small firms who, it was claimed, would be driven out of business if paid holidays were enforced by law.

Oddly enough, some of those very firms were later instrumental in pushing up wage rates and improving conditions, not because they were concerned with labour problems but because of the shortage of workers, more especially skilled workers. This was due in some degree to the effects of the second world war, when workers who were conscripted into other industries, and some who came out of the army, decided to try their luck at other types of work. However, the chief reason for the shortage of labour is due to higher education opportunities which are now within the reach of most, making possible a much wider choice of jobs and professions. Many people with whom I worked in those early days would now certainly be regarded as university material.

Some children managed to get as far as grammar school, but their parents could not afford to keep them until they were sixteen, in spite of the small education grant available at the time, so they ended up in some of those dreary, dirty workrooms I have tried to describe, with no job security, no paid holidays until 1938, no sick pay and certainly no superannuation whatever the length of service. Having mentioned grammar school places, I recall how carefully worked out were the scholarship examinations so that an elementary school with several hundred children might have an annual grammar school pass of three or four. In the early nineteen twenties I remember my father coming home from work with the following story. It appeared that the son of a very poor widow had managed to reach the finals in medicine and the entrance fee for this examination was in the region of twenty pounds. This sum was out of the question so far as the widow and her son were concerned, so a collection was organized and it was decided to ask all the various small firms round about to contribute. In this fashion the money for the finals was obtained. Such were the 'good old days' for some.

In spite of improved wages and working conditions in the fur industry, there has for years been more jobs available than people willing to do this work – especially women and girls. During the early thirties when I came out of hospital all this was very much in the future, and the competition for jobs on the lowest level was absolutely cut-throat.

Having mastered the basic elements of the work I seriously studied methods of speed which could be applied with the minimum of energy, for I was competing with other workers who were active and well. I carried out my own method of work analysis, by breaking down every movement involved in the work and examining every process. I studied all the movements and eliminated those which I thought over-extended or redundant. By this method, which proved to be more successful than anticipated, I managed to maintain a higher output of work, with the minimum amount of energy. I did not do this for medals (which workers never get anyway) but to raise my earning capacity and for my own survival. I have been teaching the trade now for many years and still try to break down the fallacy in the industry that noisy machines are synonymous with high output. Although the words sometimes addressed to me, 'You do not make much noise and never seem to be working very hard,' were not always intended as a compliment, I always took it as such, since it vindicated my system of work. What people said did not really matter because the result could be checked and the proof of the pudding was there.

As the Doctor said, 'What's five years?'

On the debit side it was a very bad thing, having to spend those years away from home, among strangers and in the highly charged atmosphere of hospitals. Bad because those formative years were spent not with the young and healthy, but with the sick and selfish. I use the word 'selfish' in this context to mean people for whom illness had disturbed the routine of their lives and whose energies were not unnaturally bent in one direction – that of getting well. Most of all, however, I suffered from loss of freedom and never came to terms with being institutionalized since by nature I am restless and impetuous.

There is also a credit side to this story. I learned to amuse and educate myself; to discipline myself to accept all manner of sudden changes. The question of sudden changes in hospital was always disturbing. Within the framework of the deadly routine, or perhaps because of it, the smallest change assumed a large significance. With the continual change-over of patients and staff, since only the ward sister was permanent, I learned to live among all kinds of people.

What's five years? Perhaps a long time in terms of pain, anxiety, frustration, loss of freedom, fear and misery; coexisting with the death of others and, by force of circumstance, compelled to watch and thereby to some extent share, the misery of others. In return for ultimate life – perhaps not very much after all.

When I say that many, many people would have wished to be me, I do not use these words in the competitive spirit of winning, because I know that the scales might have quite easily tipped the other way.